Slimming
EATS
MADE IN THE
AIR FRYER

Slimming EATS

MADE IN THE
AIR FRYER

Siobhan Wightman

Tasty recipes to save you time
– all under 600 calories

yellow
kite

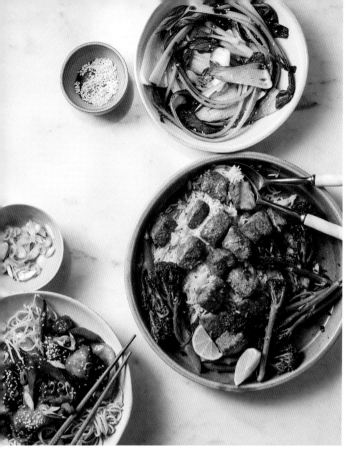
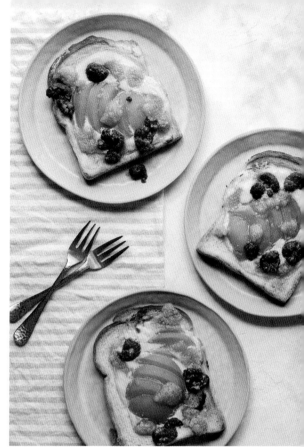
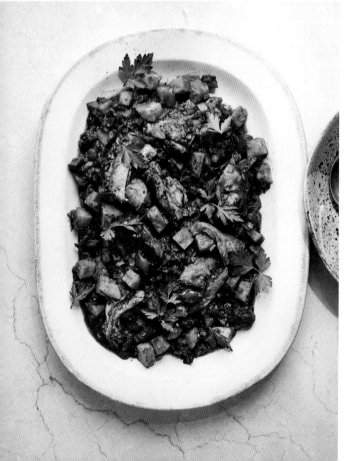
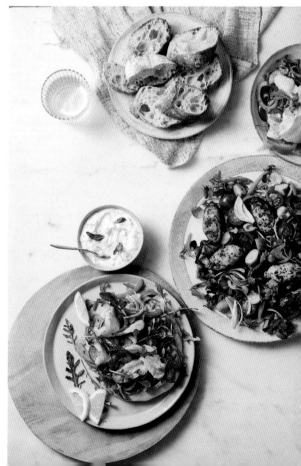

CONTENTS

HELLO!

I'm Siobhan, the creative mind and driving force behind the Slimming Eats blog and the bestselling cookbooks *Slimming Eats* and *Slimming Eats Made Simple*.

Although I was born in London, I've had the privilege of living in various places, including Ireland and different parts of England. Currently my home is in Ontario, Canada, where I have resided since 2008 with my husband and two children (my youngest was born in Canada). My Slimming Eats blog began as a personal record of my weight-loss journey, serving as a way for me to both remain accountable and share the meals I was preparing with others. I'd never have imagined where I am today with it! While on my own journey, I found that many 'low-calorie' recipes lacked taste and were overly restrictive, which wasn't inspiring, especially for families. I wanted my family to be able to enjoy the food I cooked too. Considering our busy schedules, the last thing I wanted was to have to cook separate meals.

Initially, Slimming Eats was a visual diary of my progress, and I didn't expect a large number of visitors to the website. To my surprise, however, people started leaving comments on my posts, expressing their enjoyment of my recipes and even sharing their own weight-loss achievements. The overwhelming support I received kept me motivated and inspired and it's incredible to think that I've also been able to inspire and empower so many individuals to take control of their weight-loss journey and embrace a healthier lifestyle. Through my own experience with various food regimes, I've come to understand that sustainable weight loss requires a lifestyle change, rather than a temporary diet. This philosophy underpins my recipes – I don't eliminate the foods I love or impose restrictions. Instead, I focus on cooking those foods in a healthier way and creating well-balanced meals.

As more people started following me, they encouraged me to share more content, leading to the continuous growth of Slimming Eats and a whopping following on social media (@slimmingeats). Slimming Eats has now become a full-time job that I absolutely love. I take immense pride in my unique style and recipes and live and breathe what I do!

It still feels surreal to this day to receive such love and appreciation for my recipes. My focus has always been on preparing healthy, home-cooked meals that the whole family can sit down at the table and enjoy together, chatting about their day. One thing I encourage my readers to do is to use my recipes as a base to build upon and create their own combinations. The more you cook, the more you'll learn about what works and what doesn't. This is exactly how I taught myself – by recreating my favourite foods at home in a healthier way. You can easily add variety to a simple recipe by swapping a few ingredients.

If cooking becomes fun and enjoyable for you, it will be much easier to stay motivated in the long run. I always advise taking it a day at a time and avoiding comparisons with others. Remember, this is *your* journey. Embrace healthy eating with sensible portions and make it a lifestyle change. Whether it's taking the slower, scenic route or going at a faster pace, we all share the same goal – to become healthier.

I genuinely hope you enjoy this cookbook and discover the exciting possibilities of cooking with your air fryer. Thank you so much for your continued support, which makes all of this possible.

Siobhan xx

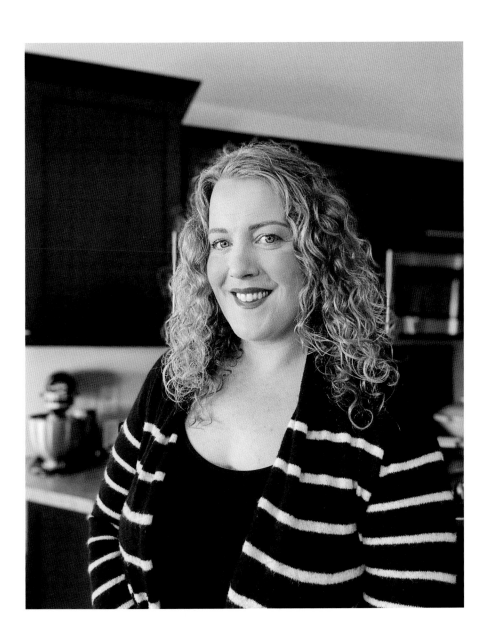

INTRODUCTION

I have to admit, writing an air fryer cookbook wasn't really on my radar at first. It hadn't even occurred to me to do such a 'specialized' book, but my publisher came to me and said, 'Everyone is going air fryer crazy. What about doing a book with just air fryer recipes?' and then members of my Facebook group were requesting the same too.

I began to think about it. An air fryer book. It seemed so limiting... and of course, as a food blogger, I already had an air fryer (and pretty much every other kitchen gadget you can think of) and I had made some air fryer recipes for my website. But a whole book – that seemed a bit restrictive and tricky! My air fryer had traditionally been used for warming things up or cooking very basic items like seasoned chicken, potatoes or fish. Could I use it, I wondered, to create lots of varied and delicious low-calorie recipes? Most of the air fryer cookbooks I had come across all seemed to be using the same kind of foods, and not really the type of foods we love as a family, which are delicious while still being low-calorie.

However, the more I thought about it, the more I decided this might be a fun challenge. What recipes could I come up with that had not been traditionally cooked in an air fryer but would save people time and even money? The more I brainstormed, the more recipes started to come out. Before long, I knew that there were going to be enough ideas for a book and I told my publisher that yes, we could do an air fryer book!

Air fryers have been gaining popularity recently for multiple reasons: they are inexpensive to buy, cheap to run and cook foods rapidly. In fact, I was amazed at just how quickly I could create these recipes when using an air fryer. Typically, when testing a recipe, I have to wait some time for it to cook and see if it has worked or not – sometimes it has, sometimes it hasn't. With an air fryer, this time is massively reduced, so I was able to test and retest recipes at a much faster pace than with a traditional recipe book. It was therefore much less stressful for me, which is always a bonus. My kids loved the testing stage of the recipes too, waiting impatiently for each recipe to come out of the air fryer so they could sample it. It was an absolute pleasure to see the delight on their faces as they tried the next new thing I made.

So there you have it – *Slimming Eats Made in the Air Fryer*. I have to say, it's been so much fun to see this book come to life and I hope it will make you love cooking in your air fryer too. I've split the book into Poultry, Pork, Lamb and Beef, Fish and Seafood, Vegetarian and Sweet Treats to keep it simple and easy to find whatever you're craving. From fakeaways to family favourites, I've included them all. And I'll let you in on a secret, I can't stop cooking in the air fryer and I think after this cookbook, you're going to fall in love with its magic too... You might never turn your oven on again!

WHAT IS AN AIR FRYER?

An air fryer is a kitchen appliance that utilizes hot air circulation to cook food, providing a healthier alternative to deep-frying. It works by using a high-powered fan to circulate hot air around the food, cooking it evenly and giving it a crispy texture without the need for large amounts of oil. The hot air is circulated by a heating element located at the top of the appliance, and the food is placed in a removable basket. The basket can be easily removed for cleaning and is usually made of non-stick material.

One of the advantages of an air fryer is its versatility. It can be used to cook a wide range of foods, from all kinds of proteins to vegetables and even desserts. Most recipes can be adapted for the air fryer by adjusting cooking times and temperatures. An oven to air fryer conversion chart can be used to help with this and I have included one on page 11. With practice, users can become adept at using their air fryer to achieve perfect results every time.

An air fryer can be a great addition to any kitchen, providing a healthier way to cook your favourite foods and a versatile cooking option for a range of recipes. When choosing an air fryer, consider the size and features that will suit your needs, and enjoy experimenting with new recipes and cooking techniques.

WHAT KIND OF AIR FRYER DO I NEED?

In contrast to a few years ago, there are now so many options for different air fryers that it can be hard to know which is the right one for you. If you are on a budget, there are some great choices available – keep an eye out for deals and sales at stores local to you as well as online. It is also worth checking out local sale groups or even thrift and secondhand stores in your area, as occasionally you can be lucky and pick up a really good deal.

Air fryers come in a variety of sizes and shapes, from small countertop models suitable for a single person or couple to larger models with multiple baskets that can cook a complete meal for a large family. When choosing an air fryer, it is important to consider the size that will suit your needs, and also the features that are important to you. Some models, for example, have additional features such as a rotisserie or dehydrator, while others have digital controls or preset cooking programmes. For the recipes in this book I used an Instant Pot Vortex, which I love because it has a solid basket. Some of the older styles tend to have a basket with holes, which limits the types of foods you can cook unless you use an insert of some kind.

WHAT SIZE AIR FRYER DO I NEED?

My Instant Pot Vortex air fryer has a 5.7 litre (6-quart) capacity. So, you will want a similar size air fryer with a solid basket, otherwise you may need to size down the recipes.

If you have a dual basket air fryer, that should be fine – you can cook the recipes using the two baskets on the match cook/dual cook mode. Dual basket air fryers are the new style of air fryer available and they are becoming hugely popular – the dual baskets are a great option, even for a small family, because it means you can cook two different things at once.

Gone are the days when you would have to cook the protein side of things in the air fryer and then use the hob for sides or additions, because with a dual air fryer you can pretty much make a complete meal for your whole family without even having to turn on the oven or hob. I do have a dual basket air fryer (in fact I have probably been through every type of air fryer that has existed), but still prefer my single basket for meals because of the large capacity basket.

The main thing you want to ensure when purchasing an air fryer is that you pick the right size for your family. A single person or small family of two may manage with a small one basket air fryer of quite small capacity – usually around 3 litres (which is up to about 1–3 quarts). However, I'd say a family of two should opt for the next size, which is 6 litres (up to 4–6 quarts). If you have a large family, you might want to invest in the large capacity models or a dual basket air fryer of 9 litres (up to 6–8 quarts in size).

I always recommend going for the biggest size you can afford and, of course, that can fit in your kitchen, because having the extra capacity when you need it will always be useful.

It really is a case of picking the type that is going to be best for you. So I recommend researching before you buy. Ask friends who already have one what model/make they have, what kind of capacity it has, and what they like or dislike about it.

CAN I COOK ANY OF THESE RECIPES IN AN ORDINARY OVEN?

The great news is that almost anything you can cook in an oven can also be cooked in an air fryer with just a few recipe modifications, and vice versa. To adjust a recipe that is not specifically designed for an air fryer, you should, as a basic rule, reduce the cooking temperature by around 25 degrees Fahrenheit (see my easy conversion chart below) and then decrease the oven cooking time by 20 per cent. Bear in mind, however, that these are only general guidelines, as all air fryers vary.

The conversion chart opposite will also help you adjust most air fryer recipes for oven cooking. Use it to guide you, though when cooking recipes from this book, please bear in mind that they have not been tested for oven cooking and results may therefore differ. As you gain experience in using your air fryer, you'll become more familiar with its cooking patterns and be able to determine the ideal temperature for different types of food.

OVEN TIME (mins)	AIR FRYER TIME (mins)
10	8
15	12
20	16
25	20
30	24
35	28
40	32
45	36
50	40
55	44
60	48

OVEN TEMP	AIR FRYER TEMP
165°C /325°F	150°C /300°F
180°C /350°F	165°C /325°F
190°C /375°F	175°C /350°F
200°C /400°F	190°C /375°F
220°C /425°F	200°C /400°F
230°C /450°F	220°C /425°F

TIPS FOR AIR FRYING

There are many different things you can do to ensure successful cooking in an air fryer, as follows;

READ THE MANUAL

While most things are pretty straightforward, I can't overstress the importance of reading the manual that comes with your air fryer and getting used to all its different features (including safety features to ensure you don't void its warranty). While most air fryers work the same, there will be differences in terms of buttons and features, and, say, what can be removed for cleaning. Try a few simple recipes first until you get the hang of cooking with it.

PREHEAT YOUR AIR FRYER

It is recommended that you preheat your air fryer for at least 2–5 minutes, especially if you want a sear/crisp to whatever you are cooking. In cases where you want, say, a steak to be nicely browned, you'll need to make sure your air fryer is nice and hot before adding it to the basket.

WATCH OUT FOR COOKING TIMES

While cooking times are usually given in recipes, these can only be a guideline as there are many different factors that can change timings, such as the brand of air fryer you use, its wattage and the thickness of the foods you are cooking, such as different cuts of meat.

CHECK THE FOOD WHEN COOKING

I always recommend checking food around the halfway mark of cooking time. That way you can adjust things if needed, especially when cooking a particular dish for the first time. If you find it is cooking too high or too low, you can adjust the temperature. This is also a great time to give things a little flip, if needed. Remember, not all air fryers will cook exactly the same – some things may need slightly longer cooking times, others slightly less.

DON'T OVERFILL THE BASKET

One of the most crucial tips for air-frying success is to avoid overcrowding the basket. Filling the basket beyond its capacity can result in uneven cooking, leaving some portions of food undercooked while others are overdone. This can lead to the undesirable outcome of the food being steamed and producing a soggy, unappetizing texture rather than the crispy exterior that air-frying is known for. So, make sure that the basket isn't overcrowded, allowing sufficient space for the hot air to circulate and cook the food evenly.

USE A LITTLE COOKING OIL

While it's possible to cook oil-free in an air fryer, using a small amount of oil can make a significant difference in achieving optimal results. Typically, just one tablespoon of oil is sufficient for a recipe intended to serve 4 people and can greatly enhance the flavour and texture of the finished dish. In some recipes, I may opt for low-calorie sprays, such as olive oil spray, but only when I'm confident that it won't compromise the overall quality of the dish.

In my experience, certain recipes truly benefit from the addition of a small amount of oil, and the extra calories are well worth it. Nevertheless, it's crucial to practice moderation and avoid excessive use of oil in any given recipe. By doing so, you can strike the ideal balance between taste and nutrition, and create delectable air-fried dishes that are both healthy and delicious.

KNOW WHEN TO USE THE GRILL PAN

A lot of air fryers come with a grill pan insert, but when should you use this? If it's a dish that is saucy or when I don't want the food to get too dry, I will remove the grill pan. (Remember, anything with liquids, like sauces/marinades etc. will drain underneath.) So really it's best for things like kebabs, steak and grilled meats etc. I don't use it for things like burgers, meatballs etc. as I find they become too dry and, if you are using all lean meats, you want to keep those juices next to the food.

MAKE SURE THERE ARE NO LOOSE MATERIALS IN THE AIR FRYER

This can be a concern, as the appliance uses hot air to cook food. Loose objects could block the fan or element, which could be dangerous. This is especially important for recipes that require foil to cover the food. Ensure that the foil is secured properly and does not move during cooking. If you're preheating the air fryer, make sure you don't leave the liner in there or it could catch fire.

CLEAN REGULARLY

It's crucial to clean your air fryer, especially the basket, after each use, to maintain its good condition. If you neglect cleaning, you may get a build-up of food particles in the basket that can be difficult to remove, and the pan may lose its non-stick coating.

MAKE SURE YOU USE NON-STICK BAKING PAPER (OR PARCHMENT PAPER)

This is important to avoid your food sticking to the paper.

EXPERIMENT WITH RECIPES

The recipes in this book demonstrate the versatility of your air fryer as they are not restricted to the usual foods that you may associate with air-frying. There really are endless possibilities. You can experiment with new recipes you find or modify your favourite recipes using the conversion chart and tips I've provided. Don't hesitate to explore and unleash your creativity with your air fryer!

AIR-FRYER ACCESSORIES

There are a wide range of accessories available for air fryers, should you choose to buy them. However, virtually any dish that is suitable for an oven is also suitable for air-frying, as long as it fits in your air fryer and doesn't obstruct the air flow or touch the heating elements.

To simplify the cleaning process, I often use non-stick baking paper and foil tray inserts in my air fryer. Additionally, a 20cm (8in.) cake barrel/tin and appropriately-sized metal skewers are essential for certain recipes, such as kebabs. If your air fryer has a smaller capacity, it may be necessary to use a smaller-sized barrel/tin or skewers.

When using foil to prevent over-browning, as in some of the recipes, it's important to ensure the foil is tightly wrapped around the container or dish to prevent it from moving around. You may also consider purchasing additional racks and silicone tray inserts, but I recommend only buying the accessories you think you'll use regularly. It's tempting to buy all the available accessories when purchasing a new gadget, but many may go unused.

SCALING DOWN RECIPES

Scaling down recipes can be an incredibly useful skill to have in your culinary repertoire. Not only does it allow you to tailor recipes to suit the size of your family or gathering, but it also helps to reduce food waste, save money, and even provide more accurate portion control.

As previously mentioned, the majority of the recipes are designed to serve four individuals, perfectly fitting the size of my family. However, if you're preparing a meal for fewer people and want to adjust the quantity accordingly, all you need to do is halve the ingredients in the recipe. While the cooking time should remain the same, it's crucial to monitor the food closely, as smaller quantities of ingredients may cook more quickly. Maintaining the correct ratio of ingredients is also important to ensure the dish remains flavourful. Therefore, always taste and add more seasoning if you think it is required. Overall, with a bit of practice and attention to detail, it's possible to create perfectly sized meals every time, regardless of their original serving size.

SLIMMING EATS INGREDIENTS

I always try to use foods that are readily available all over the world – most are storecupboard staples. There may be a couple of more unusual ingredients that add authenticity to a dish, so if you are struggling to find these, always check online for local sources, such as Asian grocers. Failing that, Amazon has most things. If you can't source a particular ingredient and have looked everywhere, Google is always great for looking for substitutions. Here are some notes about some of the ingredients I use.

DAIRY PRODUCTS

Cheese: When it comes to cheeses like Cheddar or mozzarella, I consistently choose the regular versions instead of reduced-fat options. I believe that regular cheese offers more flavour and melts better. I also prefer to buy cheese in block form and grate it myself, rather than purchasing pre-grated cheese in bags. The pre-grated cheese often has a starchy coating to prevent clumping in the bag, which can interfere with its melting capabilities.

Cream cheese: I choose the light or reduced-fat versions, although the calorie difference isn't significant in some cases. It's very important to note that cream cheese and quark are not the same thing. Cream cheese can withstand heat and create a creamy sauce without separating, while quark tends to split when heated and has a more sour taste. It is an ingredient you will see me use often in recipes to create a delicious creamy sauce that is lower in calories.

Milk: I prefer either semi-skimmed or whole milk. I'm not particularly fond of skimmed milk, due to its watery taste. If a recipe specifically calls for semi-skimmed milk, I suggest following that instruction to achieve the desired outcome. On the other hand, if you're looking for a dairy-free alternative, oat milk and cashew milk are wonderful options that are known for their creamy taste, even though they are not technically dairy products.

Reduced-fat cream alternative: Reduced-fat cream alternative is a fantastic ingredient for achieving a creamy sauce without adding excessive calories. It is typically available in both single and double cream variations, providing options for different recipe needs. This ingredient allows you to enjoy the rich and velvety texture of a creamy sauce while keeping the calorie content in check. In North America, look for what is called 'half and half' (a milk/cream blend).

Yogurts: My usual choice is fat-free Greek or plain varieties. However, if you prefer unflavoured yogurts with 2% fat, the calorie difference isn't significant. The only instance where I may opt for whole-milk yogurt is when it's needed in a recipe that involves heating, as whole-milk yogurt won't separate in sauces.

GRANULATED SWEETENER

Where granulated sweetener is used in a recipe, I always use Erythritol, which is naturally derived. I have probably used every type of sweetener there is over the years and I find this one acts and tastes the closest to real sugar in recipes. If you are choosing to use a different type of sweetener, then you must check the packaging to ensure you use the correct ratio to sugar, as provided on the packing. Otherwise it could affect the taste or your baking results. With Erythritol, I generally use it like for like with sugar, but with other types of sweetener you may need a lot less or more. If you don't like to use any sweeteners like this and prefer to just use sugar, honey or maple syrup, then of course you can definitely do this. It will just increase the calories in a recipe if you are making that swap.

HERBS AND SPICES

As regular cooks, most of us will already have a pretty good collection of dried herbs and spices. However, if you find there are some you don't have, just buy as you need it for a recipe. It can be overwhelming to go out and try and find everything at once.

HONEY AND MAPLE SYRUP

These two ingredients will work pretty much the same in any recipe. They have slightly different flavour profiles but, other than that, you can swap one for the other in any recipe as you like.

LEAN MEATS/PROTEIN

In this book, the nutritional information always focuses on lean cuts of meat as this helps keep the calorie count low. I make sure to trim any visible fat, even if the packaging claims it's lean. Sometimes boneless chicken thighs, for example, can still have significant fat attached. I find that kitchen scissors work well for trimming any visible fat.

For mince (ground meats), I prefer lean options with around 5% fat. Going any leaner can make dishes, like burgers or meatballs, a bit dry. However, you can use leaner if you prefer, especially if the meat is cooked ground or as mince, as I find this can be more versatile in recipes, especially when in a sauce.

In recipes like curries and casserole-type dishes involving chicken, you'll notice that I often tend to use thighs instead of breast meat. This is because thighs are more flavourful, add richness to the dish, and remain tender. Chicken breast tends to cook quickly and can become dry in these types of recipes. Plus it often doesn't offer the same depth of flavour.

LOW-CALORIE SPRAY

I like to use olive oil spray mostly and one that doesn't contain emulsifiers.

OLIVE OIL, BUTTER AND GHEE

For the most part, I will use low-calorie spray. However, where I feel a recipe needs it, I use a small amount of olive oil or butter. Ghee is a great ingredient for things like curries, but any cooking fat will work in its place. When eating healthy, don't be scared of using healthy cooking oils in moderation. A small amount in a meal for four won't add up to that many calories.

SALT AND PEPPER

These simple ingredients always deserve their own separate mention. They are what I call the basic flavour enhancers. Everyone has a different level of preferred seasoning and that's why it is very important to taste food as you go along and adjust the seasoning as needed.

If you use these as intended, your food will never be bland. It's a misconception that you need to add heaps of spices and heat in order to add flavour. While they do add flavour, if your food is bland, all that could be needed is a little more salt and pepper. You will be surprised at how much they will pop the flavour of something in a dish, by just adding an additional pinch to your food.

When it comes to seasoning, salt and pepper are the foundation, but don't hesitate to adjust other spices according to your taste. If you prefer spicier food, feel free to add more spice. If there's a spice or herb you dislike, it's usually fine to omit or replace it with a similar alternative, as long as it doesn't play a crucial role in the dish.

The recipes I've provided should serve as a starting point and, as you gain experience in the kitchen, you'll become more familiar with what works and what doesn't in a recipe. Please experiment and personalize the flavours to suit your preferences.

STOCK

An important thing to note about using stock in recipes is that not all stock cubes/bouillons etc. are equal. This is one of the biggest mistakes I see when a certain measurement of stock is called for in a recipe.

Different brands will require different ratios of liquid, so always check the packaging of the one you are using. For example, some stock cubes are mixed with just 180ml (6fl oz) of water, which makes 180ml (6fl oz) of stock. So, if you are only using one of those for, say, 480ml (16fl oz) of stock, it's going to be very bland and watery in taste, which can affect the whole flavour of a recipe.

Then there are other stock cubes where, if you're making over 500ml (17fl oz) of stock, and you used one of those and only mixed it with, say, 240ml (8½fl oz) of water, it would be quite salty and could overpower the recipe.

SPECIAL DIETARY REQUIREMENTS

Next to each recipe, whenever possible, you'll find dietary labels indicating whether the recipe is vegetarian, dairy-free or gluten-free. If a substitution is made to make the recipe allergen-free, please note that it may affect the final nutritional analysis, unless the original recipe already includes that ingredient.

However, it's crucial to always double-check the products and ingredients you use in any recipe to ensure they are allergen-free, as different brands may vary. While I personally use allergen-free stock, spices and condiments, it's essential for individuals with dietary requirements to carefully scrutinize all the ingredients they use.

ALLERGEN-FREE ALTERNATIVES

If you or someone you know can react to allergens, here are some excellent alternatives to day-to-day foods that may be causing you problems.

BREADCRUMBS

Opt for gluten-free versions or make your own by processing gluten-free bread that's a few days old in a food processor. It's a simple way to ensure your recipes remain gluten-free, while still enjoying the texture and crunch.

CHEESES

There is now a wide range of dairy-free cheese options available, although I haven't personally experimented with them extensively. Some varieties are more flavourful than others.

MILKS

Of the many dairy-free alternatives available, cashew milk and oat milk are my favourites. Unlike almond milk, they offer the same creamy texture as regular milk without having a pronounced nutty taste. You can even make your own easily. Coconut milk makes an excellent dairy-free substitute for creamy sauces, although, if using the light versions, you may need to add a little starch to thicken.

PASTA

Swap wheat-based pasta for gluten-free alternatives, like brown rice pasta, quinoa pasta, or chickpea pasta. There are a great variety of options available now – just make sure you follow the package directions when cooking as they can be different to regular pasta.

THICKENERS

Cornflour (cornstarch) is an excellent gluten-free choice for thickening sauces. Unlike flour, it doesn't require butter to create a roux, making it lower in calories and reducing the overall calorie content in a recipe. Arrowroot flour and tapioca starch are also gluten-free alternatives for thickening sauces. Some people prefer to use xanthan gum but, personally, I find that it can easily lead to an overly thick and gloopy sauce if used excessively.

SAUCES AND CONDIMENTS

When it comes to ingredients like soy sauce, Worcestershire sauce, hoisin sauce and others, there is now a wonderful variety of allergen-free versions available. While the flavour may vary slightly, these alternatives ensure that you no longer have to miss out on certain recipes that previously required ingredients you couldn't try. It's an exciting opportunity to explore new flavours and enjoy dishes that were previously off-limits. Coconut aminos is an excellent alternative to soy sauce, especially for individuals with soy allergies or those avoiding soy-based ingredients. In fact, there are now sauces available that traditionally use soy but are made with coconut aminos instead.

SOURCING ALLERGEN-FREE INGREDIENTS

When sourcing allergen-free sauce alternatives, there are several options available. You can find them in specialty health food stores, organic markets, or sections dedicated to allergen-free products in larger supermarkets. Additionally, many online retailers now offer a wide range of allergen-free ingredients, making it convenient to explore and purchase these products from the comfort of your own home. Don't hesitate to inquire with store staff or check reliable online resources to find the best places to obtain these allergen-free sauce or condiment options.

VEGETARIAN CHOICES

If you're looking to make some more of the recipes in this book meat-free, while still containing lots of protein, here are some swaps you can try. Please note that cooking times may vary, so some experimentation might be needed:

Beans, lentils and pulses: Substitute meat with protein-rich options like edamame, black beans, kidney beans, white beans, lentils, or pinto beans to add bulk and nutrients to your meals.

Cheese: Opt for firm cheeses such as paneer and halloumi that hold their shape well when grilled or pan-fried, providing a satisfying texture in various dishes.

Eggs: Eggs are versatile and quick sources of protein that can be prepared in a variety of ways – boiled, fried, poached, scrambled, or used in frittatas and omelettes.

High-protein pastas: Look for pasta options made from chickpeas, lentils, or similar ingredients. These pasta varieties provide additional protein to your meals.

Jackfruit: Young green jackfruit has a fibrous texture that can mimic pulled pork or shredded chicken when cooked. It works well in BBQ sandwiches, tacos, or curries. Make sure to use the unripe, canned variety in brine or water, not the ripe sweet jackfruit.

Meat substitutes: Tofu, seitan, tempeh, soya pieces (crumbles), and Quorn are excellent choices to increase protein content in your recipes.

Quinoa: Incorporate this pseudo grain, which offers a nutty flavour, as a great source of protein and fibre.

Vegetables: Roasted, sautéed, raw, or grilled, vegetables make wonderful meat substitutes. They can be used in tacos, stir-frys, curries, pasta dishes and more, adding flavour and texture to your meals. Mushrooms, especially varieties like portobello, shiitake, or oyster mushrooms, have a meaty texture and rich flavour. They are great for burgers, stir-frys, and as a topping for pizzas.

Remember to experiment with seasonings, marinades, and cooking methods to enhance the flavours and textures of these meat substitutes. Enjoy your plant-based cooking!

PORTIONS AND NUTRITIONAL INFORMATION

The nutritional information provided for each recipe in this book pertains to a single portion or serving and exclusively includes the ingredients listed in the recipe. It does not include any supplementary side dishes or serving items.

It is important to note that the portion sizes presented in the book are merely a recommendation. Individuals possess different appetites, so while a recipe may be suitable for my family of four, it may prove inadequate or excessive for others. Nevertheless, I always try to keep to the recommended servings and balance out my meals with nutritious vegetables if I find myself particularly hungry. The appropriate portion sizes and the inclusion of healthy vegetables will largely depend on your specific calorie objectives and appetite. However, if your aim is to shed weight, it is crucial to ensure that you do not exceed your daily calorie limit, as this can impede weight-loss efforts.

Rather than increasing portion sizes to make meals more substantial, a healthier approach is to incorporate additional vegetables onto your plate. There are several methods to accomplish this. For instance, you can replace a portion of carbohydrates on your plate with vegetable alternatives, such as cauliflower rice, spiralized vegetables, vegetable mash, or roasted vegetables. Alternatively, you can enhance the volume of your plate by incorporating low-calorie, nutrient-dense vegetables. Personally, I often complement my meals with a side of vegetables or a salad.

Beside each recipe, you will see dietary symbols, which state which recipes are vegetarian, gluten-free and dairy-free, plus which are freezer-friendly.

When a recipe includes the freezer icon, it can be frozen and stored in the freezer for a maximum of 3 months.

FREEZING AND STORING TIPS

Recipes suitable for freezing are marked with a freezer symbol. There really isn't much that can not be frozen – it's more to do with personal preference. For example, cooked pasta may not be enjoyable when reheated, and some sauceless dishes can become dry, especially with lean protein.

Here are some tips for freezing and storing food:

Cool the food down properly first. Before freezing any cooked food, make sure to cool it down quickly. Divide large portions into smaller containers to speed up the cooling process. This helps prevent the growth of bacteria and ensures better food quality. Rice, for example, can be safely reheated if refrigerated or frozen promptly after cooling down. Reheat it only once, ensuring it's heated thoroughly.

Use freezer-friendly packaging. Choose packaging materials that are suitable for freezing. Sturdy, airtight containers or freezer bags are ideal. Make sure they are labelled as freezer-safe to prevent freezer burn and maintain the freshness of the food. Choose containers of similar shape and size for easy stacking.

Store whole garlic bulbs in a container and peeled whole ginger too. Frozen ginger can be grated directly into recipes. Freeze chillies like Thai red chillies or jalapeños to prevent spoilage and ensure availability.

Control your portions. Freeze food in individual or meal-sized portions whenever possible. This allows for easier defrosting and helps to minimize waste.

Use protective layers. When freezing separate items like burgers or thin cuts of meat, or cake, place a layer of wax paper between each piece to prevent them from sticking together.

Organize your freezer. Arrange your freezer in a way that allows you to easily identify and access the oldest items. Move the oldest dated items to the front and the newest items to the back. This helps prevent food from getting forgotten or going bad in the freezer. You can also keep an inventory of what you have in the freezer to keep track of items and prevent food waste.

Label and date. Clearly label each container or bag with the contents and date of freezing to avoid confusion. I like to use a marker directly on the container instead of relying on labels that may fall off.

Know how to reheat properly. For optimal results, it is recommended to defrost frozen food in the refrigerator before reheating. While reheating straight from frozen is possible, using appliances such as the oven, air fryer, microwave, or hob to reheat the defrosted food generally yields better results in terms of texture and flavour.

NOW, LET'S GET COOKING!

POULTRY

GREEK TURKEY KOFTA SALAD 24

CHICKEN TACOS WITH MANGO
SALSA AND LIME CREMA 27

EASY CHICKEN PAD THAI 28

GRUYÈRE AND ASPARAGUS
STUFFED CHICKEN BREASTS 31

CHICKEN CAESAR BURGERS 32

LEMON, CHICKEN AND
ARTICHOKE BAKE 35

SOY GINGER CHICKEN 36

CHICKEN TETRAZZINI 39

HOT NASHVILLE CHICKEN WITH
CREAMY RANCH COLESLAW 40

455g (1lb) 5% fat (ground)
      turkey mince

2 garlic cloves, crushed

2 tbsp finely chopped
      fresh parsley

1 tbsp finely chopped fresh mint

1 tbsp cornflour (cornstarch)

½ tbsp honey

¼ tsp bicarbonate of
      soda (baking soda)

½ tsp salt

¼ tsp freshly ground black pepper

½ tsp dried oregano

pinch of red chilli flakes (optional)

olive oil spray

For the mint feta dip

100g (3½oz) fat-free
      Greek yogurt

100g (3½oz) feta, crumbled

1½ tbsp finely chopped fresh mint

1 garlic clove, crushed

1 tbsp lemon juice

1 tsp lemon zest

salt and freshly ground
      black pepper

1 tsp extra virgin olive oil

For the salad

100g (3½oz) mixed baby leaves

½ small red onion, finely sliced

16 Manzanilla green olives

100g (3½oz) roasted red
      peppers in brine, drained,
      rinsed and finely sliced

½ cucumber, sliced

10 cherry tomatoes, halved

GREEK TURKEY
KOFTA SALAD

1. To make the feta dip, mix all the ingredients except for the seasoning and olive oil in a bowl. Taste and season as needed with salt and black pepper. Drizzle with the olive oil.

2. Place the turkey mince in a large bowl. Add the garlic, parsley, mint, cornflour, honey, bicarbonate of soda, seasoning, oregano and chilli and mix until well combined. Spray your hands with olive oil spray and shape the mixture into 12 oval-shaped kofta patties.

3. Preheat the air fryer to 190°C/375°F for 2 minutes.

4. Line the air fryer basket with non-stick baking paper or use the grill pan insert. Add the kofta, spray over the top with olive oil spray and air-fry for 10–12 minutes until cooked. Turn the kofta halfway through cooking and spray again with olive oil spray.

5. To make the salad, place the baby leaves on a flat plate and add the red onion, green olives, roasted red peppers, cucumber and cherry tomatoes. Top with the kofta and serve with the mint feta dip.

<u>Side suggestions</u>

This salad is delicious just as it is or, for a more filling meal, served with some warmed pitta bread or rice.

<u>Variation</u>

The kofta can also be made with chicken mince.

KCALS per serving 275 FAT 12.5g SAT FAT 4.8g CARBS 12.4g SUGARS 6.7g FIBRE 2.8g PROTEIN 26.7g SALT 2.46g

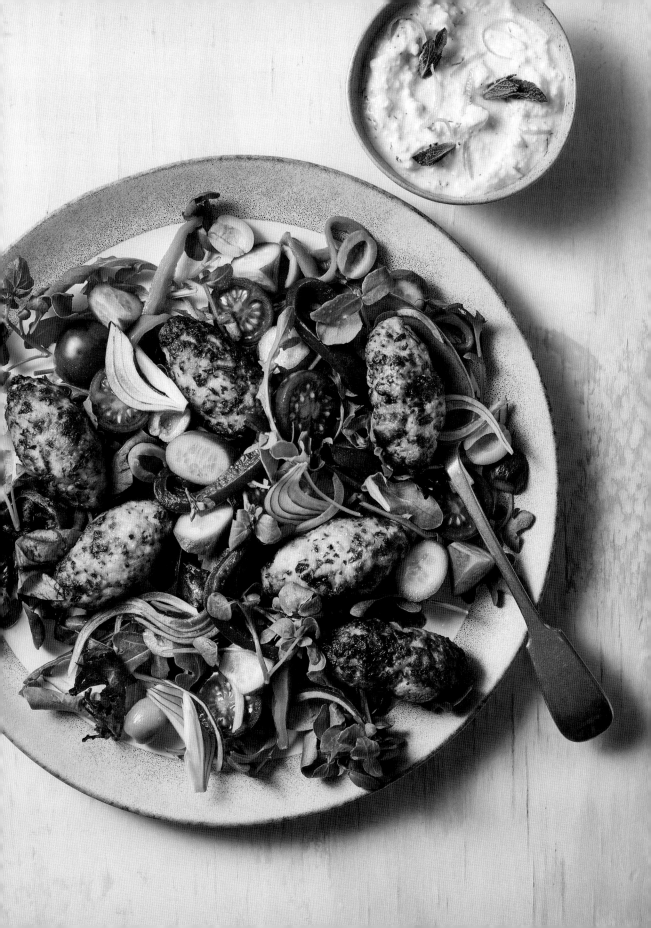

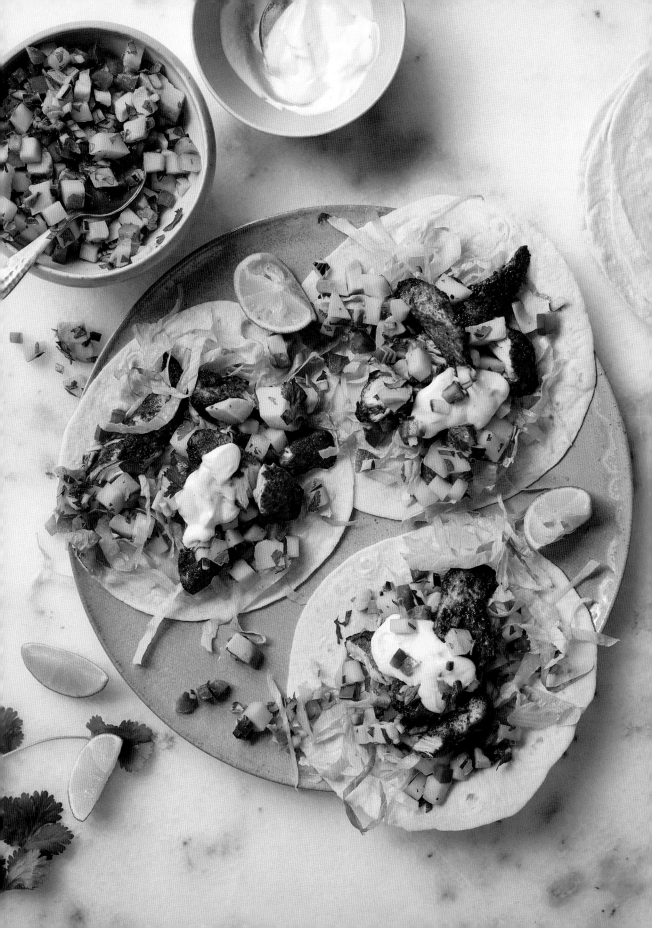

CHICKEN TACOS WITH MANGO SALSA AND LIME CREMA

500g (1lb 2oz) chicken, sliced into pieces (I use half boneless skinless chicken thighs and half chicken breast)

olive oil spray

4 low-calorie 20cm (8in.) tortilla wraps or 8 small wraps

1 romaine lettuce, shredded

For the mango avocado salsa

1 small avocado, diced

1 ripe mango, diced

¼ small red onion, diced

¼ red (bell) pepper, finely diced

1 jalapeño, seeded and diced (optional, for a bit of heat)

1 garlic clove, crushed

handful of freshly chopped coriander (cilantro)

For the lime crema

2 tbsp light mayonnaise

2 tbsp fat-free Greek yogurt

½ tsp garlic granules

salt and freshly ground black pepper

1½ tsp fresh lime juice

1 tsp granulated sweetener (optional)

For the chicken seasoning

1 tbsp sweet paprika

1 tsp garlic granules

1 tsp onion granules

1 tsp ground cumin

1 tsp mild chilli powder

½ tsp dried oregano

salt and freshly ground black pepper

2 tbsp fresh lime juice

olive oil spray

1. To make the mango avocado salsa, mix the ingredients in a bowl, season to taste and then set aside for the flavours to develop.

2. To make the lime crema, whisk all the ingredients in a jug, adding 1–2 tablespoons water to loosen the crema a little. Taste and season again if necessary. Set aside.

3. Place the chicken in a bowl with the seasoning ingredients and mix to coat well.

4. Preheat the air fryer to 190°C/375°F for 5 minutes.

5. Line the air fryer basket with non-stick baking paper or use the grill pan insert. Spray with olive oil spray, add the chicken and air-fry for 12–15 minutes until cooked through. Toss the chicken pieces halfway through cooking and spray again with olive oil spray.

6. Serve the chicken with warmed tortillas and shredded lettuce and spoon over the mango avocado salsa and lime crema.

Optional add-ons

Add a tablespoon of honey to the chicken to add a sweet-spicy flavour and help caramelization.

Swap

Swap the soft tortillas for 8 hard corn tacos.

KCALS per serving 434 FAT 12.7g SAT FAT 2.7g CARBS 37.5g SUGARS 10.9g FIBRE 12.4g PROTEIN 36.1g SALT 0.68g

300g (10½oz) boneless
  skinless chicken thighs,
  sliced into bite-sized pieces
3 garlic cloves, crushed
1 shallot, finely chopped
olive oil spray
200g (7oz) flat rice noodles
150g (5½oz) Savoy
  or Chinese leaf
  cabbage, shredded
75g (2½oz) carrot, shredded
2 eggs, beaten
pinch of freshly ground
  black pepper
125g (4½oz) beansprouts
3 spring onions
  (scallions), chopped
½ tsp red chilli flakes
  (optional)
large handful of finely
  chopped fresh
  coriander (cilantro)
2 tbsp chopped peanuts
1 lime, sliced into
  wedges, to serve

For the pad thai sauce
3 tbsp maple syrup
2 tbsp fish sauce
1 tbsp soy sauce
1½ tbsp tamarind paste

EASY CHICKEN
PAD THAI

1. To make the pad thai sauce, mix all the ingredients in a small bowl and set aside.

2. Preheat the air fryer to 200°C/400°F for 2 minutes.

3. Place the chicken, garlic and shallots directly into the air fryer basket or use a foil/silicone liner that fits. Spray with olive oil spray and air-fry for 5 minutes until the chicken is lightly golden. Turn the chicken halfway through cooking and spray again with olive oil spray.

4. Add the noodles to a bowl and cover completely with boiling hot water. Leave to soak for about 5 minutes until cooked.

5. Reduce the air fryer temperature to 190°C/375°F. Add the cabbage and carrot and air-fry for a further 3 minutes.

6. Push the chicken and veg to one side of the air fryer pan, add in the beaten eggs with a pinch of black pepper over the top and cook for 2–3 minutes, stirring halfway until the egg is just cooked (don't overcook).

7. Add in the beansprouts, spring onions and noodles along with the pad thai sauce and red chilli flakes (if using) and mix to coat.

8. Spread out the mixture in the air fryer pan and air-fry for a further 2 minutes.

9. Serve topped with coriander and chopped nuts, with lime wedges for squeezing on the side.

Tip
Tamarind paste can vary in strength and tanginess so you may need to experiment with the quantity until you achieve the desired effect. Add to the noodles a little at a time until you're happy.

Optional add-ons
You can also add some cooked prawns to this dish.

KCALS per serving 438 FAT 8.6g SAT FAT 2.1g CARBS 60.4g SUGARS 15.8g FIBRE 4.3g PROTEIN 27.6g SALT 2.97g

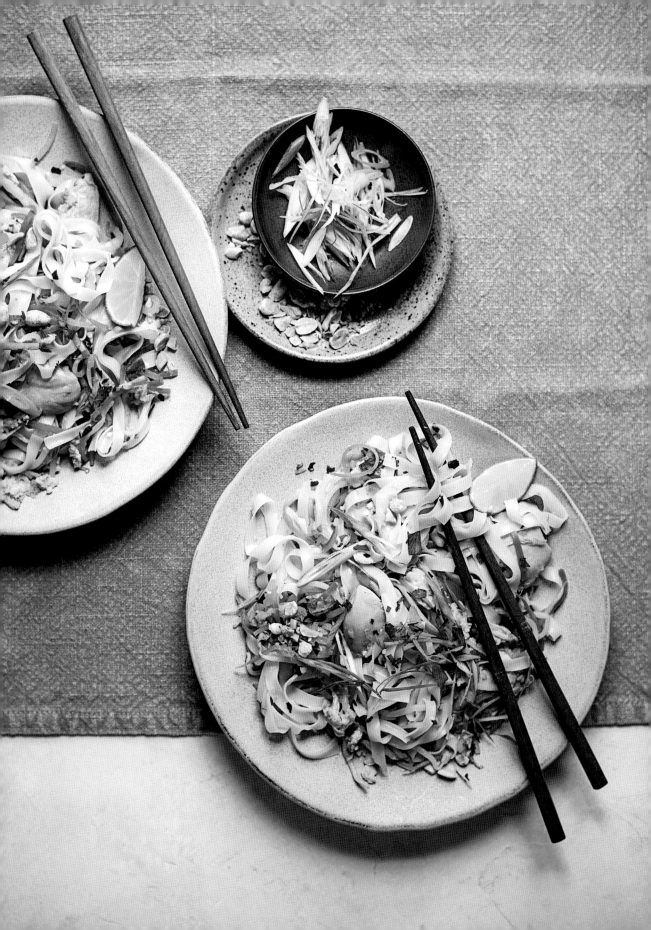

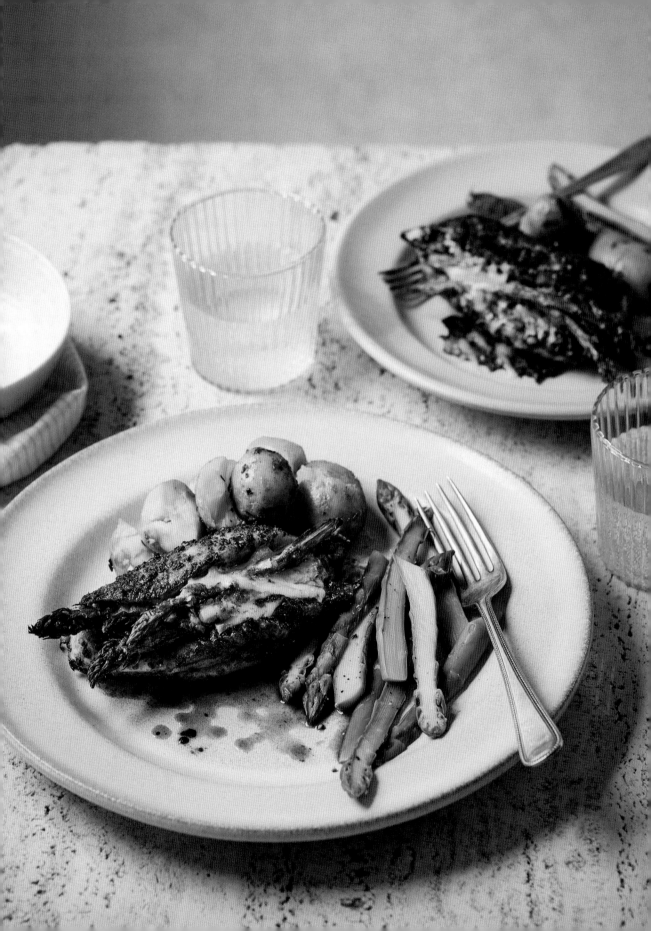

GRUYÈRE AND ASPARAGUS STUFFED CHICKEN BREASTS

4 boneless, skinless chicken
 breasts (approx. 180g each)
olive oil spray
4 tbsp tomato purée (paste)
½ tbsp maple syrup
1 garlic clove, crushed
½ tsp sweet paprika
12 asparagus spears,
 woody end trimmed
120g (4¼oz) Gruyère,
 thinly sliced

For the seasoning

1½ tsp sweet paprika
1 tsp Italian herb seasoning
1 tsp garlic granules
1 tsp onion granules
1 tsp sea salt
½ tsp freshly ground
 black pepper

1. Using a sharp knife, cut a slit down the thicker side of the chicken breasts to make a pocket.

2. Mix all the seasoning ingredients together in a bowl.

3. Spray the chicken breasts all over with olive oil spray and then rub the seasoning all over the chicken, ensuring it is completely covered.

4. Mix the tomato purée with the maple syrup, garlic and paprika and spoon this into the pocket of each chicken breast, making sure it is evenly spread inside.

5. Add 3 asparagus spears into each pocket (a small part of the stem and tip can be sticking out), then stuff each pocket with equal amounts of the Gruyère cheese.

6. Preheat the air fryer to 190°C/375°F for 2 minutes.

7. Place the chicken pockets directly in the air fryer basket (or line the basket with non-stick baking paper and spray with olive oil spray). Air-fry for 18–22 minutes until cooked (the thickest part should read 74°C/165°F when cooked).

Side suggestions

This is great served with rice, pasta, potatoes or a salad.

Swaps

*Swap the Gruyère for another flavourful cheese
of your choice, such as mature Cheddar.*

KCALS per serving 353   FAT 12.5g   SAT FAT 6.9g   CARBS 5.3g   SUGARS 4.4g   FIBRE 2.5g   PROTEIN 53.5g   SALT 2.03g

CHICKEN CAESAR BURGERS

2 large boneless, skinless chicken breasts (500g/1lb 2oz total weight)

1 tbsp cornflour (cornstarch)

1 medium egg, beaten

For the Caesar mayo

2 tbsp light mayonnaise

2 tbsp fat-free Greek yogurt

1 garlic clove, crushed

1 tbsp fresh lemon juice

1 tsp Worcestershire sauce

1 tsp Dijon mustard

2 tsp finely grated Parmesan

salt and freshly ground black pepper

For the breadcrumb seasoning

60g (2oz) panko breadcrumbs

1 tsp sweet paprika

¾ tsp garlic granules

¾ tsp onion granules

pinch of salt and freshly ground black pepper

To serve

4 small low-calorie ciabattas (I use Schär gluten-free ones) or low-calorie burger buns

a few romaine lettuce leaves, torn in half

4 x 12g (½oz) Parmesan shavings

olive oil spray

1. Slice the chicken breasts in half, cover them with cling film and flatten them with a tenderizer so you have 4 rough burger shapes.

2. Remove the cling film and lay the breasts flat on a plate. Sprinkle half the cornflour over the top, then turn them over and sprinkle the remaining cornflour over the other side.

3. To make the Caesar mayo, mix all the ingredients in a small bowl and set aside in the fridge.

4. When ready to air-fry the burgers, mix the breadcrumbs with the seasoning ingredients in a wide, shallow bowl. Place the beaten egg in another shallow bowl and then dip each chicken piece first in the beaten egg and then in the breadcrumb seasoning, tossing to coat.

5. Preheat the air fryer to 200°C/400°F for 2 minutes.

6. Line the air fryer basket with non-stick baking paper or use the grill pan insert. Spray with olive oil spray. Add the breaded chicken and spray over the top with more olive oil spray.

7. Cook for 10–12 minutes (or until burgers are cooked through). Turn the burgers halfway through and spray again with olive oil spray.

8. While the burgers are cooking you can lightly toast your ciabatta or burger buns (if you prefer) on a pan over a medium heat.

9. Remove the burgers from the air fryer.

10. Spread some Caesar mayo over the bottom ciabatta. Add the lettuce, then the burgers, then the Parmesan shavings and finally top with the other half of the ciabatta.

Note

If you prefer, the chicken can also be cooked unbreaded. Add the chicken to a bowl with 1 tbsp olive oil, 1 tsp paprika, ¾ tsp each of garlic and onion granules, ½ tsp dried oregano and salt and black pepper. Cook in the air fryer for 10 minutes on 200°C/400°F, flipping halfway through.

Optional add-ons

Add a slice of lean cooked bacon to each burger.

KCALS per serving 439 FAT 11.5g SAT FAT 4g CARBS 37.7g SUGARS 4.1g FIBRE 4.5g PROTEIN 43.8g SALT 1.52g

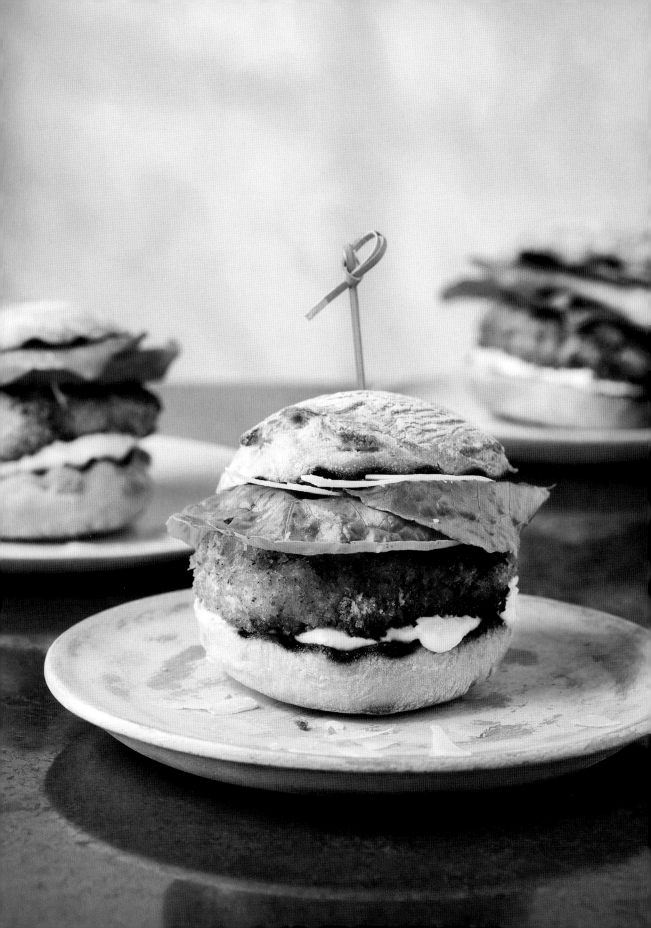

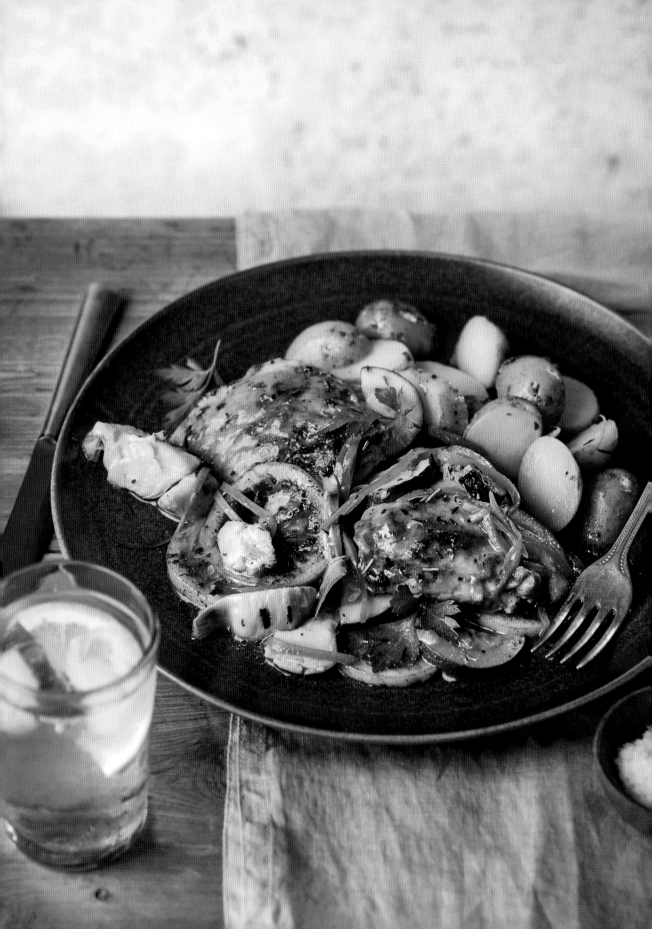

SERVES 4
PREP: **10 MINS**
COOK: **22 MINS**

8 boneless skinless, chicken thighs, trimmed of visible fat (approx. 600g/1lb 5oz total weight)

salt and freshly ground black pepper

½ tsp onion granules

½ tsp garlic granules

1 small onion, halved and thinly sliced

olive oil spray

½ jar marinated artichokes, drained

3 garlic cloves, crushed

¾ tsp dried rosemary

pinch of dried thyme

160g (5¾oz) courgettes (zucchini), halved lengthways and sliced

80g (2¾oz) carrot, shredded

1 tbsp cornflour (cornstarch)

240ml (8½fl oz) hot chicken stock

1 lemon, sliced

2 tbsp finely chopped fresh parsley

LEMON, CHICKEN AND ARTICHOKE BAKE

1. Preheat the air fryer to 200°C/400°F for 2 minutes.

2. Season the chicken thighs. Mix the onion and garlic granules together with a good pinch of salt and pepper and coat the chicken with this seasoning all over.

3. Place the thighs with the onion directly into the air fryer basket or use a foil/silicone liner that fits. Spray over the top with olive oil spray and air-fry for 6 minutes. Turn the chicken after 3 minutes of cooking.

4. Add the artichokes, garlic, rosemary, thyme, courgette and carrots and arrange around the chicken.

5. Mix the cornflour with a little water to make a slurry and combine this with the hot stock. Pour this in too and make sure the veg are all submerged in the stock (so they don't burn). Air-fry for 16 minutes, adding the lemon slices on top for the last couple of minutes.

6. Serve sprinkled with fresh parsley.

Side suggestions

This is delicious served with rice or potatoes.

Optional add-ons

Add a little grated fresh Parmesan.

KCALS per serving 241   FAT 6.5g   SAT FAT 1.6g   CARBS 9.2g   SUGARS 3.5g   FIBRE 3.5g   PROTEIN 34.6g   SALT 1.33g

SOY GINGER CHICKEN

600g (21oz) boneless,
  skinless chicken thigh
  (trimmed of visible fat),
  sliced into pieces

1½ tbsp cornflour (cornstarch)

½ tsp bicarbonate of
  soda (baking soda)

3 tbsp light soy sauce

2 tbsp dark soy sauce

2 tbsp Shaoxing wine

3 tbsp honey

2 garlic cloves, minced

5 slices fresh ginger
  6mm (¼ in.) thick

2 tsp sesame oil

200g (7oz) mushrooms,
  halved (quarter if really big)

4 spring onions
  (scallions), chopped

1. Place the chicken in a large bowl. In a jug, mix ½ tablespoon cornflour with the bicarbonate of soda and 1 tablespoon water. Pour this mixture over the chicken and mix well to coat, then set aside while you prep everything else.

2. In a jug, place the light and dark soy sauces, 100ml (3½fl oz) water, Shaoxing wine, honey, garlic, ginger, sesame oil and the remaining cornflour and whisk together until well combined.

3. Preheat the air fryer to 190°C/375°F for 2 minutes.

4. Place the chicken and mushrooms directly into the air fryer basket or use a foil/silicone liner that fits. Pour in the sauce and air-fry for 15 minutes until the chicken is cooked through and the sauce has thickened.

5. Sprinkle with the chopped spring onion and serve.

Swaps

You can use chicken breast if you prefer.

KCALS per serving 274   FAT 5.9g   SAT FAT 1.5g   CARBS 21g   SUGARS 15.1g   FIBRE 0.8g   PROTEIN 33.7g   SALT 3.27g

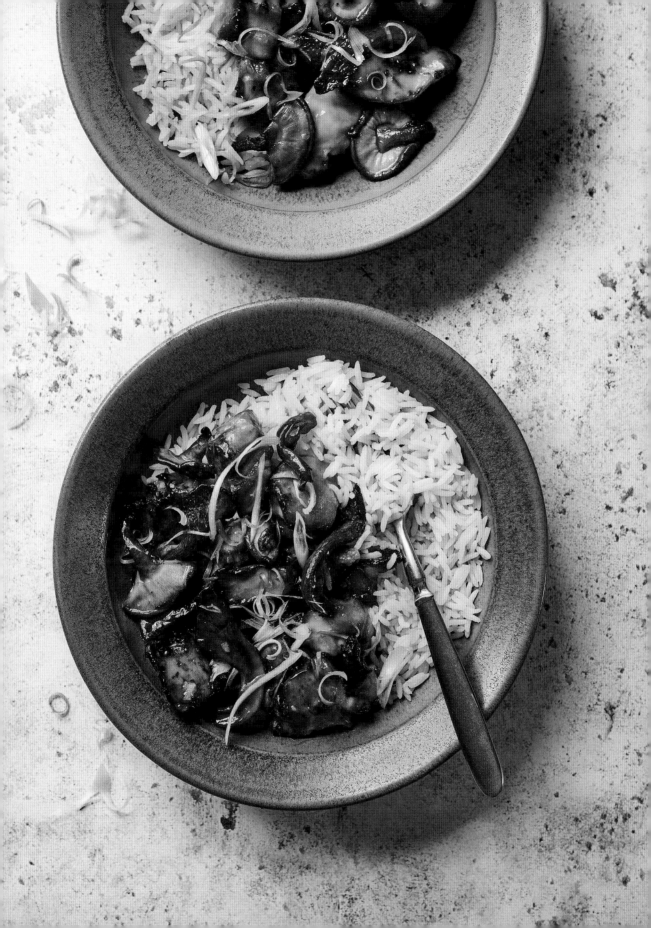

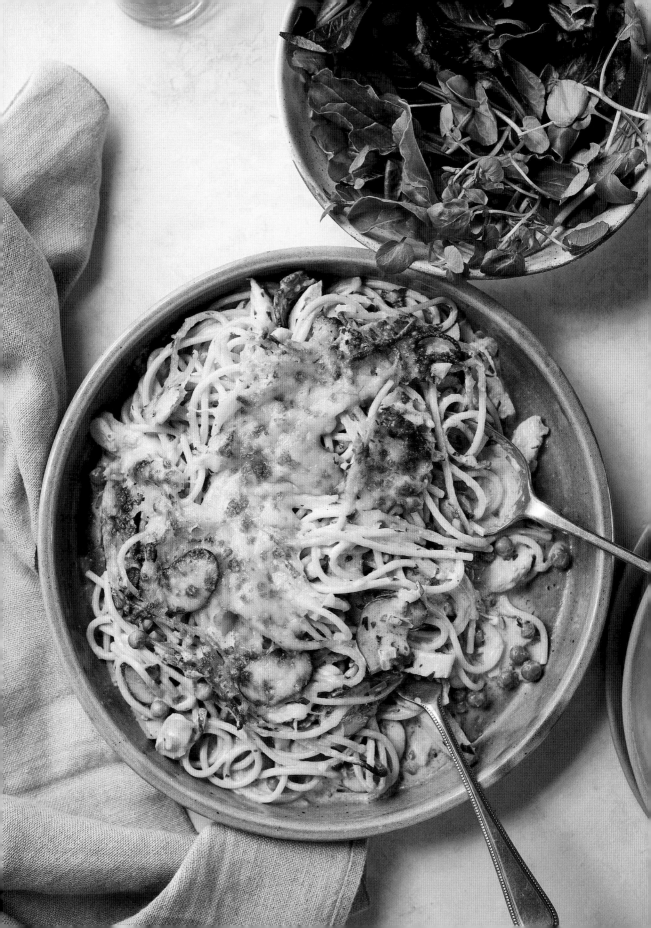

CHICKEN TETRAZZINI

1 small onion, diced

olive oil spray

250g (9oz) dried spaghetti

450g (1lb) boneless,
skinless chicken breast
(trimmed of visible fat),
sliced into large strips

salt and freshly ground
black pepper

200g (7oz) mushrooms,
thinly sliced

2 garlic cloves, crushed

2 tsp butter, melted

120g (4¼oz) light
cream cheese

180ml (6fl oz) hot
chicken stock

180ml (6fl oz) semi-
skimmed milk

2 tbsp finely chopped
fresh parsley

½ tsp garlic granules

½ tsp onion granules

80g (2¾oz) frozen peas

50g (2oz) mozzarella, grated

50g (2oz) Cheddar, grated

Tip

*If you prefer, everything
from step 9 onwards can be
completed in a 20cm (8in.)
cake barrel in the air fryer.*

1. Preheat the air fryer to 190°C/375°F for 2 minutes.

2. Place the onion directly into the air fryer basket or use a foil/silicone liner that fits. Spray with olive oil spray and air-fry for 5 minutes.

3. Cook the pasta according to the packet instructions until al dente. Reserve 80ml (2¾fl oz) of the pasta cooking water and set aside. Drain the pasta and spray with olive oil spray (this will prevent the pasta from sticking together). Toss to coat and set aside.

4. Season the chicken generously on both sides with salt and black pepper.

5. Place the chicken directly into the air fryer basket (or use a foil/silicone liner that fits) and scatter the mushrooms and garlic in between. Drizzle the melted butter over the top.

6. Air-fry for 10 minutes until cooked. Turn the chicken halfway through cooking.

7. Remove the chicken and shred it into small pieces, then add it back to the basket with the mushrooms.

8. Whisk the cream cheese in a jug with the hot stock until fully melted. Add in the milk, parsley, garlic granules and onion granules and stir until combined.

9. Combine the cooked spaghetti with the chicken mixture and add the frozen peas.

10. Pour over the cream cheese sauce along with half of the reserved pasta water and flatten down in the air fryer basket.

11. Air-fry for 4–5 minutes on 190°C/375°F until the sauce is creamy and just coats the chicken and vegetables (you can add the rest of the reserved pasta water to loosen, if necessary). Sprinkle the mozzarella and Cheddar over the top and air-fry for a couple more minutes, just until the cheese is melted and lightly golden.

KCALS per serving 548   FAT 13.7g   SAT FAT 7.5g   CARBS 54.9g   SUGARS 7.8g   FIBRE 5g   PROTEIN 48.9g   SALT 1.08g

SERVES 4
PREP: **15 MINS**
COOK: **18 MINS**

HOT NASHVILLE CHICKEN WITH CREAMY RANCH COLESLAW

8 boneless skinless chicken thighs, trimmed of visible fat (approx. 650g/23oz)

gherkin (pickle) juice for marinating

1 tbsp cornflour (cornstarch)

1½ tbsp sweet paprika

1½ tsp garlic granules

1½ tsp onion granules

1 tsp dried basil

½ tsp cayenne pepper

½ tsp dried oregano

½ tsp dried parsley

½ tsp black pepper

5 tbsp hot sauce (I used Frank's Red Hot)

2 tbsp maple syrup

sliced gherkins (pickles), to serve

For the creamy ranch coleslaw

300g (10½oz) cabbage, shredded

120g (4¼oz) carrot, shredded

1 tsp garlic granules

1 tsp onion granules

salt and freshly ground black pepper

1 tbsp gherkin (pickle) juice

2 tsp dried dill

1 tsp dried parsley

1 tsp dried chives

2 tsp sweetener

4 tbsp fat-free plain natural yogurt

4 tbsp light mayonnaise

1. Arrange the chicken in a dish in a single layer. Pour over the juice from a jar of gherkins until fully covered and marinate overnight.

2. Before cooking the chicken, place all the coleslaw ingredients in a large bowl and toss together, then set aside.

3. Drain the chicken pieces, pat dry and place in a bowl. Sprinkle with the cornflour, herbs and spices and toss until completely coated. Spray both sides of the chicken with olive oil spray.

4. Preheat the air fryer to 190°C/375°F for 2 minutes.

5. Line the air fryer basket with non-stick baking paper or use the grill pan insert. Spray with olive oil spray. Add the chicken pieces and air-fry for 16 minutes until cooked through. Carefully turn the chicken halfway through cooking and spray again with olive oil spray.

6. Mix together the hot sauce and maple syrup, then brush the chicken all over with this mixture and air-fry for a couple more minutes until cooked through and sticky with the glaze on the outside.

7. Serve with the ranch coleslaw and slices of gherkins (pickles).

Side suggestions

Additional sides include corn on the cob, mashed potato and fries. Alternatively, serve in burger buns with the coleslaw and gherkins.

Swaps

If you prefer, you can use all yogurt for a lighter coleslaw, but the mayonnaise is worth it.

KCALS per serving 369   FAT 11.9g   SAT FAT 2g   CARBS 25.6g   SUGARS 17.1g   FIBRE 6.1g   PROTEIN 36.8g   SALT 1.47g

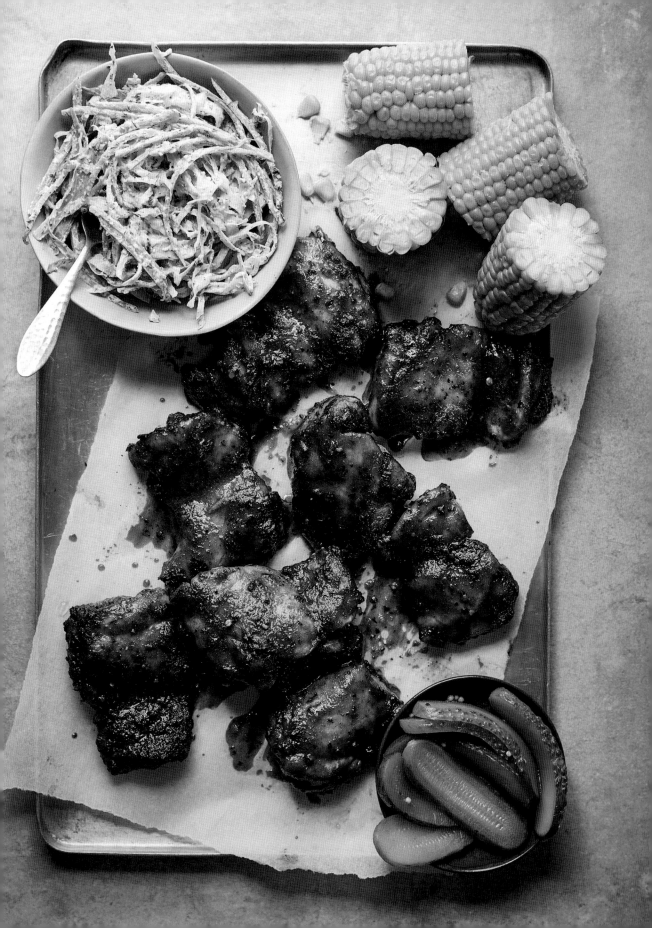

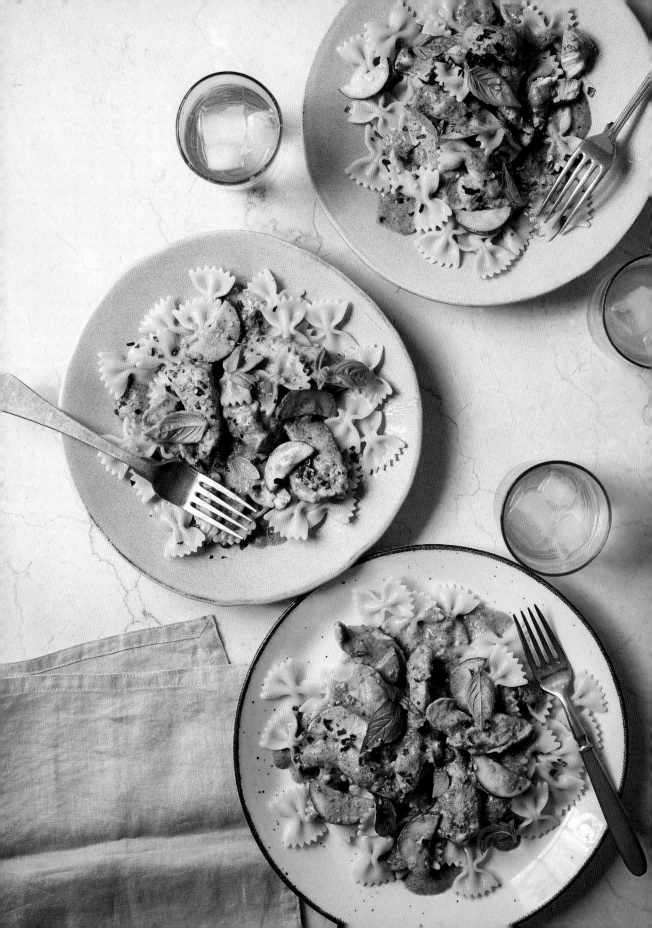

CREAMY RED PESTO CHICKEN

500g (1lb 2oz) boneless, skinless chicken breast, trimmed of visible fat and sliced into strips

1 tsp sweet paprika

1 tsp Italian herb seasoning

salt and freshly ground black pepper

olive oil spray

100g (3½oz) light cream cheese

200ml (7fl oz) hot chicken stock

4 tbsp reduced-fat red pesto

200g (7oz) canned chopped tomatoes (or 200g/7oz) fresh cherry tomatoes, halved

4 garlic cloves, crushed

pinch of red chilli flakes (optional)

1 tsp sugar (or sweetener)

160g (5¾oz) courgettes (zucchini), halved lengthways and sliced

handful of fresh basil leaves

1. Preheat the air fryer to 190°C/375°F for 2 minutes.

2. Toss the chicken in the paprika and herbs. Season with salt and pepper and spray all over with olive oil spray.

3. Add the chicken directly to the air fryer basket or use a foil/silicone liner that fits. Air-fry for 6 minutes until cooked. Turn the chicken halfway through cooking and spray again with olive oil spray. Remove and set aside.

4. Add the cream cheese to the hot stock and whisk until fully melted. Stir in the red pesto, then set aside.

5. Add the tomatoes to the air fryer basket with the garlic and chilli (if using) and a pinch of sugar. Scatter over the courgettes.

6. Pour in the sauce and air-fry for 5 minutes.

7. Add the chicken back in and continue to air-fry for another 5 minutes, until the sauce thickens.

8. Scatter with fresh basil leaves.

Side suggestions
Serve with rice, potatoes or pasta.

KCALS per serving 230   FAT 6.2g   SAT FAT 1.7g   CARBS 6.2g   SUGARS 3.9g   FIBRE 1.9g   PROTEIN 36.4g   SALT 0.81g

TURKISH CHICKEN KEBABS WITH ORZO PILAF

600g (1lb 5oz) skinless, boneless, chicken thighs (trimmed of visible fat), diced into chunks

6 tbsp fat-free Greek yogurt

1 tsp sweet paprika

1 tsp sumac

1 tsp dried mint

¾ tsp ground cumin

¼ tsp ground cinnamon

3 garlic cloves, crushed

1 tsp salt

½ tsp freshly ground black pepper

1 tbsp lemon juice

For the garlic sauce

2 tbsp light mayonnaise

3 tbsp fat-free Greek yogurt

1 garlic clove, crushed

a little lemon juice to loosen the sauce

pinch of salt

½ tbsp finely chopped fresh parsley

For the pilaf

1 tbsp butter

200g (7oz) dried orzo

1 small onion, diced

360ml (12fl oz) hot chicken stock

2 garlic cloves, crushed

To serve

lemon wedges

chopped tomatoes

sliced red onion

cucumber

1. Place the chicken in a bowl with the yogurt, herbs, spices, garlic, seasoning and lemon juice. Toss until coated, then marinate for at least a couple of hours or overnight.

2. To make the garlic sauce, mix all the ingredients in a bowl until well combined, then set aside.

3. To make the pilaf, place a 20cm (8 in.) cake barrel in the air fryer basket and preheat at 200°C/400°F for 2 minutes. When hot, add the butter and heat until melted.

4. Add the orzo and onion and air-fry for 2 minutes until the orzo is brown and toasted.

5. Add in the stock, garlic and a pinch of salt and pepper and air-fry for 23–25 minutes, stirring halfway through, until the stock is completely absorbed and the orzo is cooked (don't worry if it is still a little al dente). Remove the cake barrel, cover tightly with foil and set aside.

6. Thread the marinated chicken onto metal skewers. Alternatively, if you don't have skewers, line the air fryer basket with non-stick baking paper or use the grill pan insert. Spray with olive oil spray and place the chicken on top.

7. Air-fry the chicken for 15 minutes until cooked. Turn it halfway through cooking and spray again with olive oil spray.

8. Serve the chicken with the orzo pilaf and garlic sauce, lemon wedges, tomatoes, red onion and cucumber.

KCALS per serving 489   FAT 12.4g   SAT FAT 3.8g   CARBS 44.1g   SUGARS 5.9g   FIBRE 3.6g   PROTEIN 48.5g   SALT 2.64g

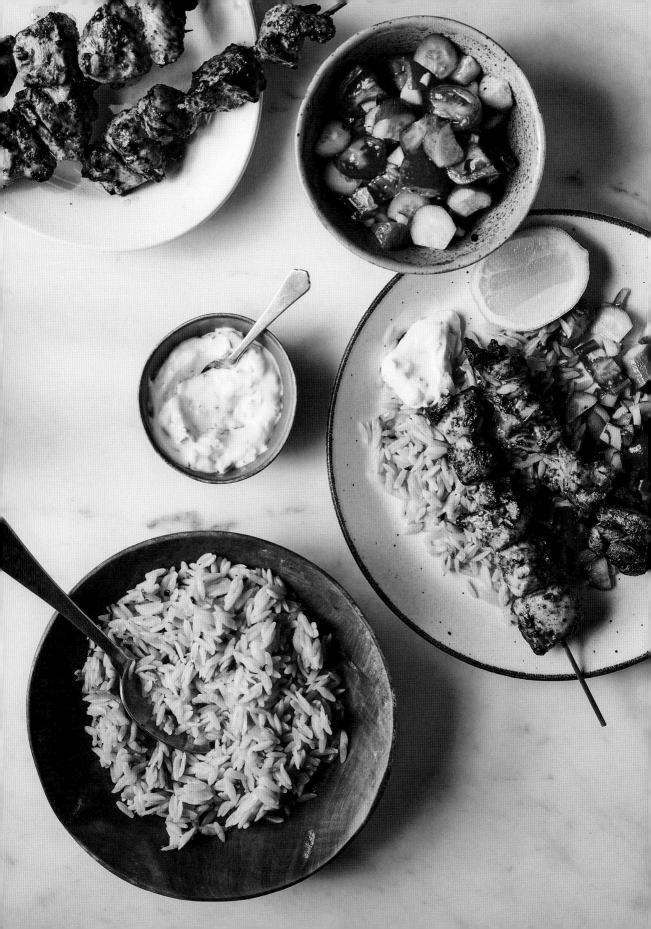

SERVES 4

PREP: **15 MINS**

COOK: **42 MINS**

500g (1lb 2oz) 5% fat turkey mince

handful of finely chopped
    fresh coriander (cilantro)

2 garlic cloves, crushed

1 tsp freshly grated ginger

1 tbsp tomato purée (paste)

¼ tsp bicarbonate of soda
    (baking soda)

pinch of red chilli flakes

½ tsp salt

½ tsp ground cumin

½ tsp ground coriander

½ tsp garam masala

olive oil spray

For the tikka masala sauce

1 tbsp ghee or oil of choice

1 onion (100g/3½oz), finely chopped

3 garlic cloves, crushed

1 thumb-sized piece of fresh
    ginger, peeled and grated

2 tsp ground cumin

2 tsp ground coriander

2 tsp garam masala

2 tsp sweet paprika

1 tsp chilli powder (or to taste)

1 tsp ground turmeric

2 bashed cardamom pods

1 tsp fenugreek leaves, optional

400g (14oz) passata

2 tbsp tomato purée (paste)

1 tbsp maple syrup

240ml (8½fl oz) hot chicken stock

120ml (4fl oz) reduced-fat
    single cream alternative

squeeze of fresh lemon juice

freshly chopped coriander (cilantro)

TURKEY TIKKA MASALA MEATBALLS

1. Place the turkey mince in a large bowl. Add the coriander, garlic, ginger, tomato purée, bicarbonate of soda, chilli flakes, salt and spices.

2. Spray your hands with olive oil spray and shape the meat into 20 meatballs.

3. Line the air fryer basket with non-stick baking paper or use the grill pan insert. Spray with olive oil spray. Add the meatballs and air-fry for 8–10 minutes at 200°C/400°F until cooked through, turning halfway through. Remove and set aside on a plate. Reduce the air fryer temperature to 190°C/375°F.

4. To make the tikka masala sauce, add the ghee to a 20cm (8in.) cake barrel and preheat in the air fryer for 2 minutes. Add the onion, garlic and ginger and air-fry for 5 minutes until lightly golden.

5. Add the spices with a couple of tablespoons of water and mix until you have a paste. Air-fry for a further minute.

6. Add in the passata, tomato purée, maple syrup and stock and stir to combine. Air-fry for 10 minutes.

7. Stir in the cream, then add the meatballs back in (along with any juices), and turn to coat in the sauce. Air-fry for 5–6 minutes.

8. Add a squeeze of fresh lemon juice and serve sprinkled with fresh coriander.

Note

The maple syrup helps to balance all the flavours of the spices in the curry. If you would prefer to use less, add gradually to your preferred taste.

Side suggestions

Serve with some basmati rice or, for a low-carb side dish, some cauliflower rice.

KCALS per serving 357   FAT 19g   SAT FAT 8.7g   CARBS 16.3g   SUGARS 12.2g   FIBRE 5.1g   PROTEIN 27.8g   SALT 1.65g

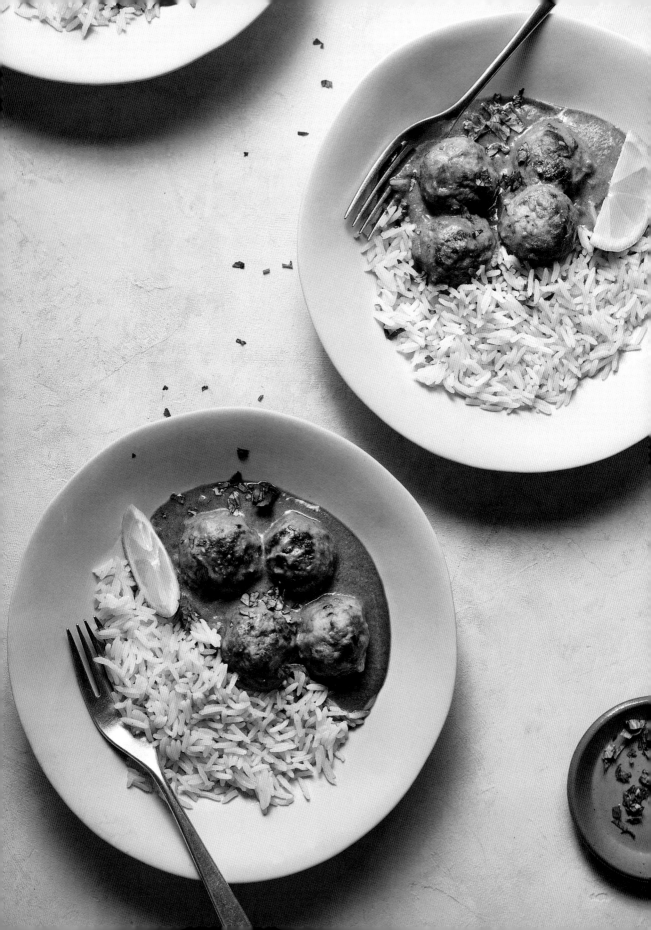

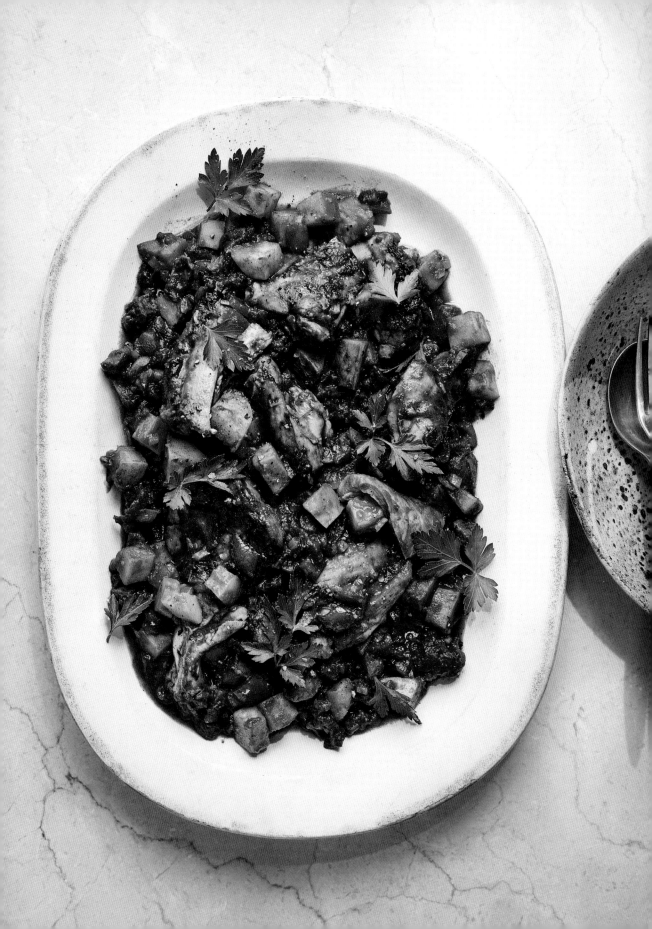

SPANISH CHICKEN, CHORIZO AND POTATO BAKE

500g (1lb 2oz) boneless, skinless chicken thighs (trimmed of visible fat), halved

2 tsp sweet paprika

1 tsp smoked paprika

1 tsp ground cumin

1 tsp ground coriander

¼ tsp ground turmeric

½ tsp onion granules

½ tsp garlic granules

salt and freshly ground black pepper

½ tsp dried oregano

pinch of red chilli flakes

For the bake

400g (14oz) potatoes, diced (I leave the skins on, but you can peel if you prefer)

½ tbsp extra virgin olive oil

3 garlic cloves, crushed

1 onion, diced

½ green (bell) pepper, diced

½ yellow (bell) pepper, diced

½ red (bell) pepper, diced

salt and freshly ground black pepper

80g (2¾oz) chorizo, diced

200g (7oz) good-quality canned plum tomatoes

100g (3½oz) passata

2 tbsp tomato purée (paste)

150ml (5fl oz) hot chicken stock

2 tsp granulated sweetener

olive oil spray

finely chopped fresh parsley or coriander (cilantro), to serve

1. Preheat the air fryer to 190°C/375°F for 2 minutes.

2. To prepare the bake, place the potato directly in the air fryer basket in a single layer or use a foil/silicone liner that fits. Drizzle with the olive oil and cook for 5 minutes.

3. Add the garlic, onion, (bell) peppers and a pinch of salt and pepper. Air-fry for 10–15 minutes until the onions and peppers are softened and lightly browned and the potatoes are fork-tender. Shake halfway through and add the chorizo.

4. Place the chicken in a large bowl. Add all the seasonings and toss to coat, then set aside.

5. Pour the plum tomatoes into a jug and crush into smaller pieces. Add the passata, tomato purée, stock and granulated sweetener and stir to combine.

6. Pour the sauce into the air fryer and stir to distribute evenly. Nestle the seasoned chicken thighs into the sauce (the top of the chicken thighs should be above the sauce) and spray over the top with olive oil spray.

7. Air-fry for an additional 16–18 minutes until the chicken is cooked through and the sauce has thickened. (Brush the chicken with the sauce halfway through cooking to prevent any burning on top.)

8. Serve sprinkled with fresh parsley or coriander.

KCALS per serving 391   FAT 13.8g   SAT FAT 4g   CARBS 28.6g   SUGARS 9.8g   FIBRE 7g   PROTEIN 34.5g   SALT 1.44g

550g (1lb 4oz) boneless, skinless chicken thighs, trimmed of any visible fat and chopped into bite-sized pieces

½ tsp garlic granules

½ tsp onion granules

½ tsp ground ginger

pinch of salt and white pepper

2½ tbsp cornflour (cornstarch)

olive oil spray

½ onion, chopped

½ red (bell) pepper, chopped

½ yellow (bell) pepper, chopped

50g (1¾oz) sugar snap peas, halved

chopped spring onions (scallions) and sesame seeds, to serve

For the sauce

2 tbsp light soy sauce

1½ tbsp tomato ketchup

½ tbsp hoisin sauce

2 tbsp honey

1 tbsp rice vinegar

1 tsp sesame oil

2 garlic cloves, crushed

½ tbsp freshly grated ginger

½ tsp red chilli flakes

½ tbsp cornflour (cornstarch)

GENERAL TSO CHICKEN

1. Pat the chicken dry with paper towels.

2. Place the chicken in a bowl with the garlic granules, onion granules, ground ginger, salt and white pepper and cornflour and toss to coat.

3. Preheat the air fryer to 200°C/400°F for 2 minutes.

4. Line the air fryer basket with non-stick baking paper or use the grill pan insert. Spray with olive oil spray. Add the chicken pieces and space as far apart as you can. Spray over the top with more olive oil spray.

5. Air-fry for 15 minutes, turning after 10 minutes and removing the baking paper, if using (this will ensure the chicken goes really crispy). Remove the chicken and set aside in a small ovenproof dish.

6. Add the onion, (bell) peppers and sugar snap peas, spray with oil and air-fry for 5–6 minutes until tender. Shake the basket halfway through cooking.

7. Place all the sauce ingredients in a microwave-proof bowl along with 4 tablespoons water and microwave at 30-second intervals, stirring after each 30 seconds until thickened (this will probably take 2 minutes in total). Alternatively, heat the sauce in a small saucepan.

8. Pour the sauce over the chicken and toss to coat.

9. Add the chicken back in the air fryer for a minute or two, just to rewarm. Sprinkle with the chopped spring onion and a pinch of sesame seeds. Serve with the vegetables.

Side suggestions

This is delicious with rice or noodles for a great fakeaway night.

KCALS per serving 271   FAT 6.2g   SAT FAT 1.3g   CARBS 27.2g   SUGARS 14.8g   FIBRE 2g   PROTEIN 25.7g   SALT 1.72g

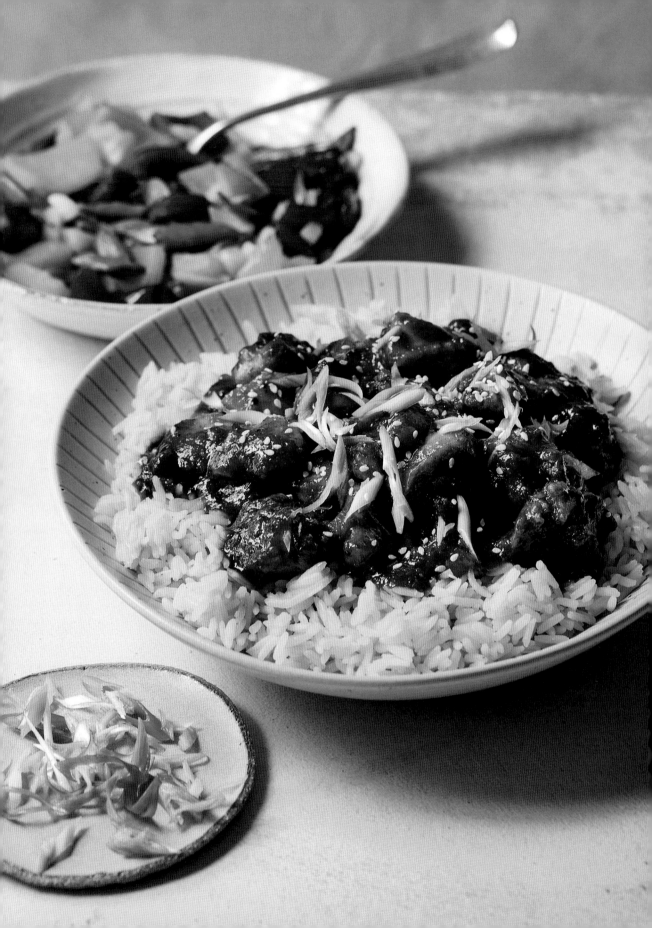

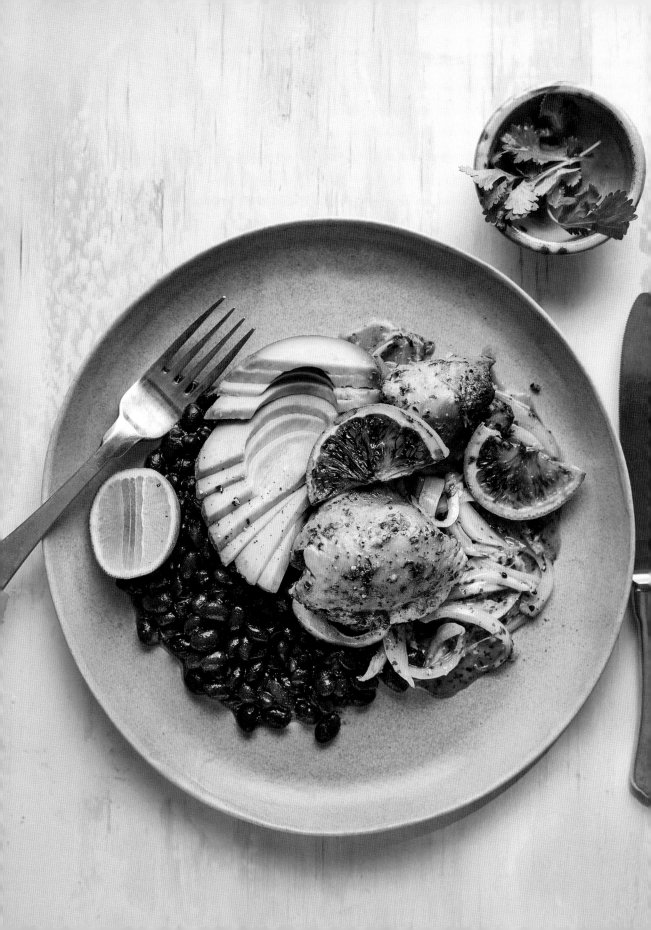

CUBAN MOJO CHICKEN

8 boneless, skinless chicken thighs, trimmed of visible fat (approx. 650g/23oz)

1 onion, quartered and thinly sliced

120ml (4fl oz) hot chicken stock

olive oil spray

3 orange slices, halved

salt and freshly ground black pepper

small handful of chopped fresh coriander (optional), to serve

For the marinade

handful of finely chopped fresh coriander (cilantro)

1 tbsp finely chopped fresh mint

1 tbsp extra virgin olive oil

4 garlic cloves, crushed

1½ tsp ground cumin

1 tsp salt

¾ tsp dried oregano

½ tsp freshly ground black pepper

1 tsp orange zest

6 tbsp fresh orange juice

3 tbsp fresh lime juice

1. To make the marinade, blitz all the ingredients in a food processor or blender until well combined. Pour over the chicken, toss to coat and then place in the fridge overnight.

2. Preheat the air fryer to 190°C/375°F for 2 minutes.

3. Place the chicken thighs along with any leftover marinade directly into the air fryer basket or use a foil/silicone liner that fits. Scatter the onion in between the chicken.

4. Pour the stock in between the chicken thighs, ensuring the onion is submerged in the stock.

5. Season the top of the chicken thighs with a pinch of salt and black pepper and spray over the top with olive oil spray. Air-fry for 16–18 minutes until the chicken is cooked through. Halfway through, spoon some of the sauce over the top of the chicken. Add the orange slices for the last 3 minutes.

6. Scatter with some fresh coriander, if using, and serve.

Side suggestions

This is delicious served with white rice, black beans and avocado.

KCALS per serving 245 FAT 9.4g SAT FAT 1.9g CARBS 6.2g SUGARS 4.8g FIBRE 1.6g PROTEIN 33g SALT 2.04g

250g (9oz) dried pasta
   of your choice

olive oil spray

450g (1lb) boneless, skinless
   chicken breast (trimmed of
   visible fat), sliced into strips

1 onion, thinly sliced

3 slices of lean bacon
   medallions, finely chopped

salt and freshly ground
   black pepper

2 ripe tomatoes (250g), finely
   diced, seeds and core removed

For the chicken seasoning

2 tsp sweet paprika

1 tsp smoked paprika

1 tsp onion granules

1 tsp garlic granules

salt and freshly ground
   black pepper

For the sauce

4 tbsp tomato purée (paste)

240ml (8½fl oz) chicken stock

½ tbsp balsamic vinegar

1 tbsp brown granulated sweetener

2 garlic cloves, crushed

½ tbsp dark soy sauce

1 tsp Worcestershire sauce

For the topping

50g (1¾oz) Monterey Jack
   or Cheddar, grated

50g (1¾oz) Red Leicester or
   Double Gloucester, grated

2½ tbsp barbecue sauce
   (use a good-quality one
   for best flavour)

3 spring onions (scallions), sliced

MONTEREY CHICKEN PASTA BAKE

1. Cook the pasta according to the packet instructions until al dente. Reserve 60ml (4 tablespoons) of the pasta cooking water and set aside. Drain the pasta and spray with olive oil spray (this will prevent the pasta from sticking together). Toss to coat and set aside.

2. Preheat the air fryer to 190°C/375°F.

3. To make the seasoning, mix all the ingredients together in a bowl until well combined. Toss the chicken in the seasoning and spray all over with olive oil spray.

4. Place the onion directly into the air fryer basket or use a foil/silicone liner that fits). Arrange the chicken on top.

5. Make a little space at the side of the chicken and add the bacon. Air-fry for 6 minutes until cooked, turning halfway through.

6. Remove the chicken and roughly slice up into shreds, then place back in the air fryer. Remove three-quarters of the bacon and set side.

7. To make the sauce, whisk the tomato purée, stock, balsamic vinegar, sweetener, garlic, soy sauce and Worcestershire sauce together in a jug. Pour the sauce over the chicken and air-fry for 5 minutes.

8. Stir in the pasta with half the fresh tomato and the reserved pasta water.

9. Top with the grated cheeses and scatter over the reserved bacon. Air-fry at 180°C/350°F for approximately 8 minutes, until the cheese is melted and lightly golden.

10. Drizzle with the barbecue sauce and scatter with the remaining tomato and sliced spring onion.

Side suggestions

Serve with a mixed salad or some green vegetables of your choice.

KCALS per serving 578   FAT 14.6g   SAT FAT 6.9g   CARBS 60.2g   SUGARS 11.3g   FIBRE 6.9g   PROTEIN 48.1g   SALT 1.91g

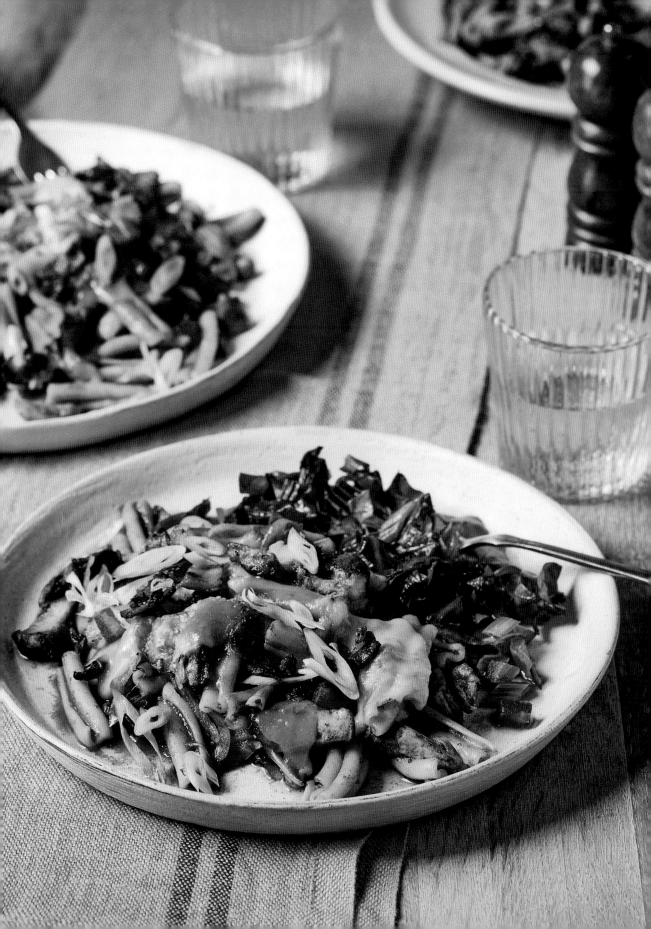

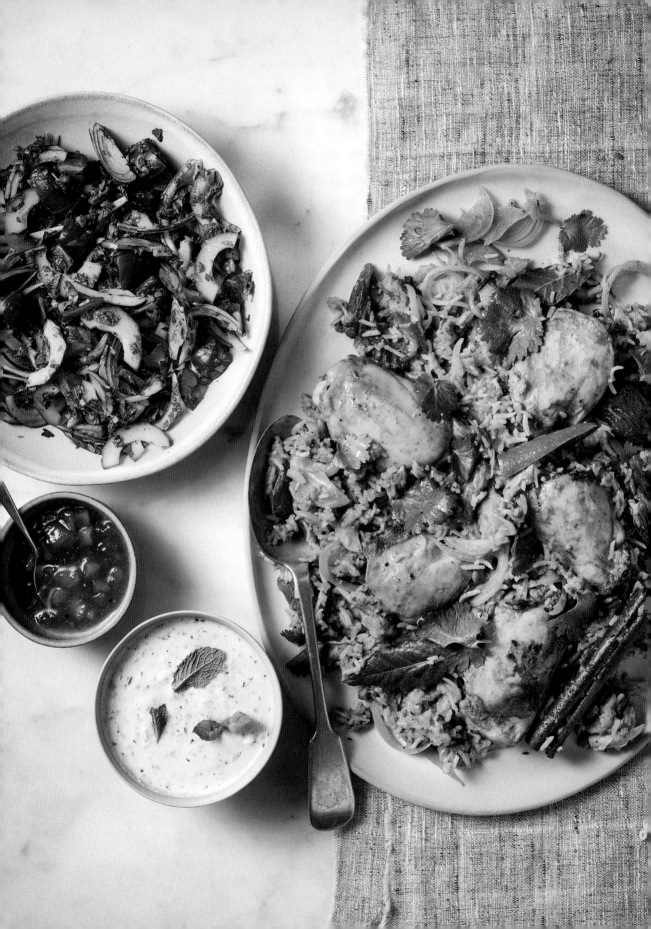

INDIAN CHICKEN AND TURMERIC RICE

600g (1lb 5oz) skinless, boneless chicken thighs (trimmed of visible fat), halved

6 tbsp plain fat-free yogurt

1 tbsp tomato purée (paste)

4 garlic cloves, crushed

1 tbsp grated fresh ginger

1 tbsp lemon juice

1 tbsp honey

1 tsp chilli powder (medium or hot according to preference)

2 tsp ground cumin

2 tsp ground coriander

1 tbsp curry powder

1 tsp garam masala

1 tsp dried mint

½ tsp ground turmeric

1 tsp salt

pinch of freshly ground black pepper

100g (3½oz) onion, thinly sliced

olive oil spray

8 baby roma tomatoes, halved

handful of chopped fresh coriander (cilantro), to serve

For the turmeric rice

180g (6½oz) basmati rice

1 tsp ground turmeric

1 tsp cumin seeds

3 cloves

4 cardamom pods

1 tbsp butter, melted, or ghee

480ml (16¼fl oz) hot chicken stock

1 whole cinnamon stick

2 bay leaves

1–2 green chillies, sliced in half

1. Place the chicken in a bowl with the yogurt, tomato paste, garlic, ginger, lemon juice, honey, spices and seasoning and mix until thoroughly coated. Set aside to marinate in the fridge for at least 30 minutes, or overnight.

2. Preheat the air fryer to 200°C/400°F for 2 minutes.

3. Place the onion in a 20cm (8 in.) cake barrel and layer the chicken pieces on top so that the onion is fully covered. Spray over the top with olive oil spray and air-fry for 8–10 minutes until the chicken is a nice golden colour on top.

4. While the chicken is cooking, place the rice in a bowl with the spices and melted butter or ghee and toss until everything is coated and the rice is flecked yellow from the turmeric.

5. Scatter the tomatoes in between the chicken and distribute the rice on top in an even layer. Spray over the top with olive oil spray and air-fry for 1 minute, until it goes almost translucent.

6. Pour in the hot chicken stock, making sure it covers everything, and nestle the cinnamon bark, bay leaves and green chilli into the rice.

7. Cover tightly with foil (this is important), then place the cake barrel back in the air fryer and air-fry for 25 minutes. Turn off the air fryer and leave to sit for 2–3 minutes before you remove the foil.

8. Scatter with fresh coriander to serve.

Side suggestions

Serve with some fat-free plain yogurt and an Indian salad made from 1 small red onion, halved and thinly sliced, ½ cucumber, finely chopped, 1 ripe tomato, cored, deseeded and finely chopped, and mixed with 1 tbsp finely chopped fresh mint, 1 tbsp finely chopped fresh coriander, a pinch of salt and pepper and a squeeze of lemon or lime juice.

KCALS per serving 464   FAT 11.7g   SAT FAT 3.8g   CARBS 46.6g   SUGARS 11.6g   FIBRE 4.9g   PROTEIN 40.7g   SALT 2.8g

PORK

WARM BACON, HALLOUMI,
SWEET POTATO AND
CHICKPEA SALAD 62

SAUSAGE, BEANS, TOMATO
AND EGG TART 65

CHINESE FIVE SPICE PORK
WITH FRIED RICE 66

HAM AND BRUSSELS SPROUTS
BUBBLE AND SQUEAK CAKES 69

CHEDDAR PESTO EGGS WITH
POTATOES AND BACON 70

HONEY AND MUSTARD SAUSAGES
WITH BUTTERNUT SQUASH 73

SMOKED ST LOUIS BBQ
PORK STEAKS 74

SAUSAGE AND GNOCCHI BAKE 76

THAI GREEN PORK CURRY 79

GARLIC BREAD SAUSAGE ROLLS
WITH MARINARA SAUCE 81

CARAMELIZED
VIETNAMESE PORK 82

PORK WITH RICH MUSHROOM
AND ONION GRAVY 85

BACON, CHEDDAR AND
SWEETCORN FRITTERS 86

CAJUN PORK WITH SWEET
POTATO AND APPLE 89

CUMIN-ROASTED PORK STEAKS
WITH GARLIC GREEN BEANS 90

MINI 'NDUJA PORK BURGERS
WITH FENNEL, TOMATOES AND
SEASONED POTATO WEDGES 93

DETROIT-STYLE
SUPREME PIZZA 94

SERVES 4
PREP: 15 MINS
COOK: 35 MINS

WARM BACON, HALLOUMI, SWEET POTATO AND CHICKPEA SALAD

150g (5½oz) canned chickpeas, drained and rinsed

½ tbsp extra virgin olive oil

1 tsp sweet paprika

¼ tsp garlic granules

¼ tsp onion granules

salt and freshly ground black pepper

olive oil spray

4 slices of lean bacon, chopped

100g (3½oz) mixed baby greens

For the sweet potatoes

250g (9oz) sweet potato, peeled and cubed

½ tbsp extra virgin olive oil

½ tsp sweet paprika

½ tsp garlic granules

pinch of salt

1 tbsp cornflour (cornstarch)

For the honey, balsamic tomatoes and halloumi

1 tbsp honey

1 tbsp balsamic vinegar (aged is best)

2 garlic cloves, crushed

½ tsp Italian herb seasoning

250g (9oz) cherry tomatoes, halved

200g (7oz) halloumi, cubed (approx. 16 pieces)

½ small red onion, very finely sliced

1. Preheat the air fryer to 200°C/400°F for 2 minutes.

2. Toss the chickpeas in the olive oil, paprika, garlic granules, onion granules and salt and pepper.

3. Line the air fryer basket with non-stick baking paper and spray with olive oil spray. Spread the chickpeas out on the paper and air-fry for 10 minutes. Turn the chickpeas halfway through cooking.

4. While the chickpeas are cooking, toss the sweet potato in the olive oil, paprika and garlic granules, with a pinch of salt. Sprinkle with the cornflour and toss to coat.

5. Once the chickpeas are golden and crisp, remove and set aside.

6. Add the sweet potato cubes and air-fry at 190°C/375°F for about 15 minutes until golden and tender. Set aside.

7. To make the honey, balsamic tomatoes amd halloumi, mix the honey, balsamic vinegar and crushed garlic cloves in a jug. Add a pinch of salt and black pepper and the Italian herb seasoning and toss the cherry tomatoes in the dressing.

8. Arrange the tomatoes with the dressing in the air fryer in a single layer and scatter the halloumi in between. Air-fry for 10 minutes at 200°C/400°F until the tomatoes are all softened and the halloumi is golden. Scatter in the red onion for the last 2 minutes and spoon over some of the sauce from the tomatoes.

9. Cook the chopped bacon according to your favourite method.

10. Arrange the baby leaves in a large oval plate, scatter with the chickpeas, sweet potato cubes, roasted tomatoes, halloumi, bacon and red onion slices and drizzle with the sauce from the tomatoes (this is the salad dressing). Dig in and enjoy!

KCALS per serving 399   FAT 19.2g   SAT FAT 9.9g   CARBS 30.8g   SUGARS 15.1g   FIBRE 6.8g   PROTEIN 22.3g   SALT 2.3g

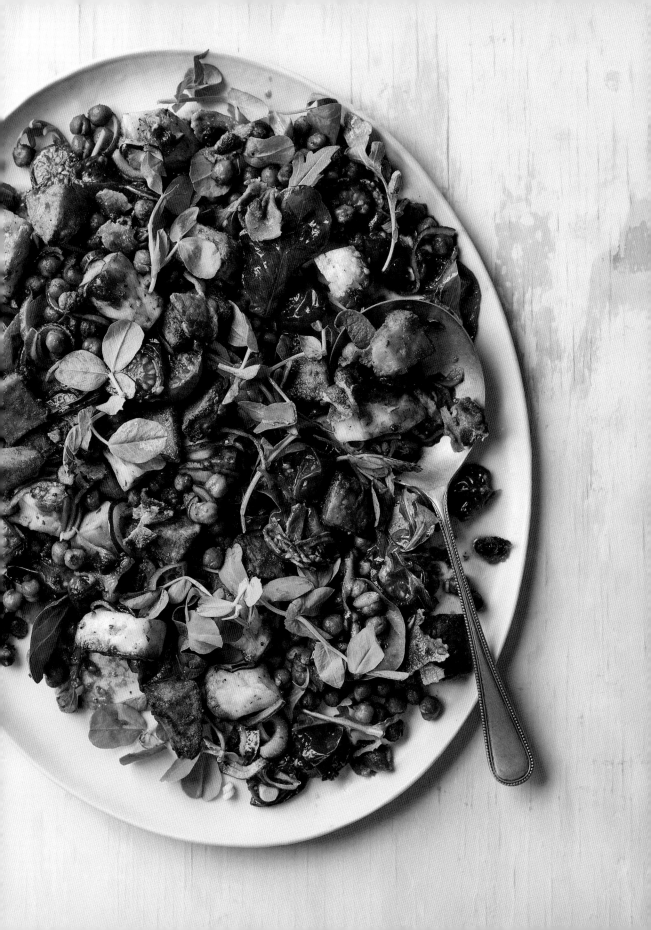

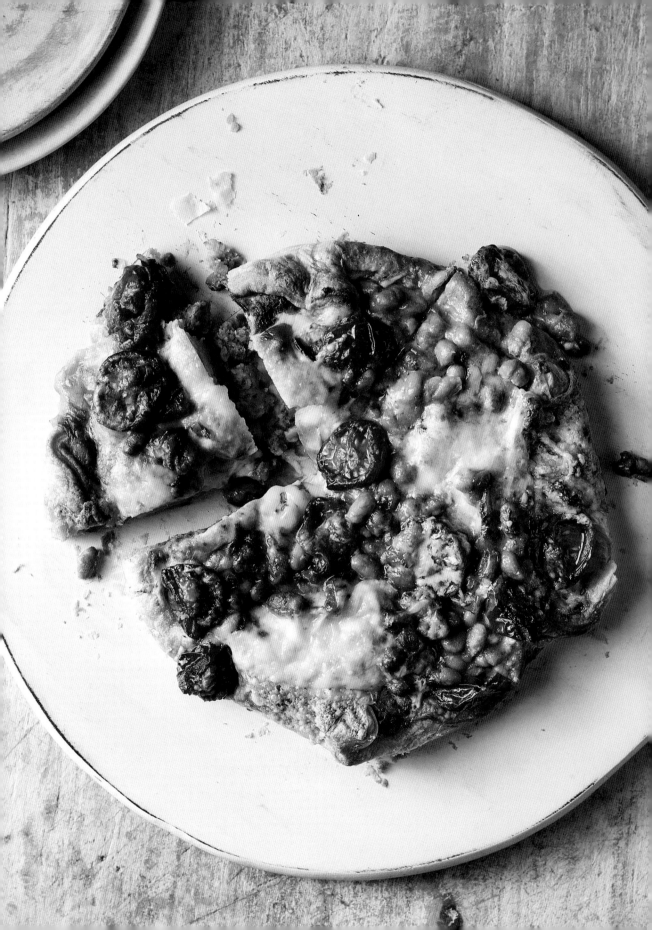

SERVES 4
PREP: **10 MINS**
COOK: **12 MINS**

SAUSAGE, BEANS, TOMATO AND EGG TART

200g (7oz) ready-rolled
   square of reduced-
   fat puff pastry

4 reduced-fat sausages
   (approx. 120g/4¼oz),
   skin removed

olive oil spray

4 eggs

100g (3½oz) canned baked
   beans in tomato sauce

6 cherry tomatoes halved

60g (2oz) Cheddar, grated

salt and freshly ground
   black pepper

1. Preheat the air fryer to 190°C/375°F for 2 minutes.

2. Lay out the pastry on a flat surface and add the sausage meat to the pastry in 4 circles (these will be the wells to crack in your eggs and keep them in place).

3. Line the air fryer basket with non-stick baking paper and spray with olive oil. Add the sausage-topped pastry and air-fry for 5 minutes until the sausage is almost cooked.

4. Remove the pastry and, using a large spoon, squash down the half-cooked sausage-topped pastry circles. Carefully crack the eggs into the circles (you can roll the edges of the pastry slightly over the egg to keep them in place), then add the baked beans and tomatoes, roughly scattered. Season with a pinch of salt and pepper, spray over the top with olive oil spray and air-fry for a further 5–6 minutes until the eggs have cooked.

5. Scatter over the Cheddar and air-fry for a further 2 minutes until the cheese is melted and golden. Season with a pinch of salt and black pepper.

6. Slice and enjoy!

Note

The cheese can be omitted, if you prefer.

Tip

Wondering what to do with the unused 120g (4¼oz) pastry from your 320g (11oz) pack? Check out the Cinnamon Sugar Twists with Dark Chocolate Drizzle on page 199.

KCALS per serving 365   FAT 20.1g   SAT FAT 9.7g   CARBS 26g   SUGARS 2.9g   FIBRE 2.7g   PROTEIN 18.7g   SALT 1.44g

200g (7oz) beansprouts

175g (6oz) mushrooms, thinly sliced

1 small onion, finely diced

2 garlic cloves, crushed

1 thumb-sized piece of fresh ginger root, thinly sliced

olive oil spray

455g (1lb) 5% fat pork mince (ground pork)

100g (3½oz) cabbage (Savoy or Chinese), shredded

60g (2oz) carrot, sliced into thin matchsticks

195g (6½oz) uncooked white rice (I like to use short grain for this, but basic long grain is fine too), precooked and chilled overnight

2 tbsp Shaoxing wine

2 tbsp dark soy sauce

1 tbsp light soy sauce

1 tbsp oyster sauce

1 tsp Chinese five spice

1 star anise

1 tbsp honey or maple syrup

pinch of freshly ground black pepper

3 spring onions (scallions), sliced

CHINESE FIVE SPICE PORK WITH FRIED RICE

1. Rinse the beansprouts with cold water and set aside.

2. Preheat the air fryer to 200°C/400°F for 2 minutes.

3. Place the mushrooms, onion, garlic and ginger directly into the air fryer basket or use a foil/silicone liner that fits. Spray with olive oil spray and cook for 3 minutes.

4. Add in the pork, cabbage and carrot and air-fry for 5 minutes. Turn the pork halfway through cooking and give it a stir.

5. Add in the rice, Shaoxing wine, soy sauces, oyster sauce, Chinese five spice, star anise, honey and seasoning and mix everything together until the pork and vegetables are evenly coated in the sauce. Stir in the beansprouts and cook for a further 3 minutes.

6. Sprinkle with the sliced spring onion and serve.

Optional add-ons

This is delicious topped with a fried egg.

Note

The cooked ratio of rice equals approx. 400g (14oz).

KCALS per serving 389   FAT 6.5g   SAT FAT 2.2g   CARBS 49.8g   SUGARS 8.7g   FIBRE 3.3g   PROTEIN 31.3g   SALT 2.32g

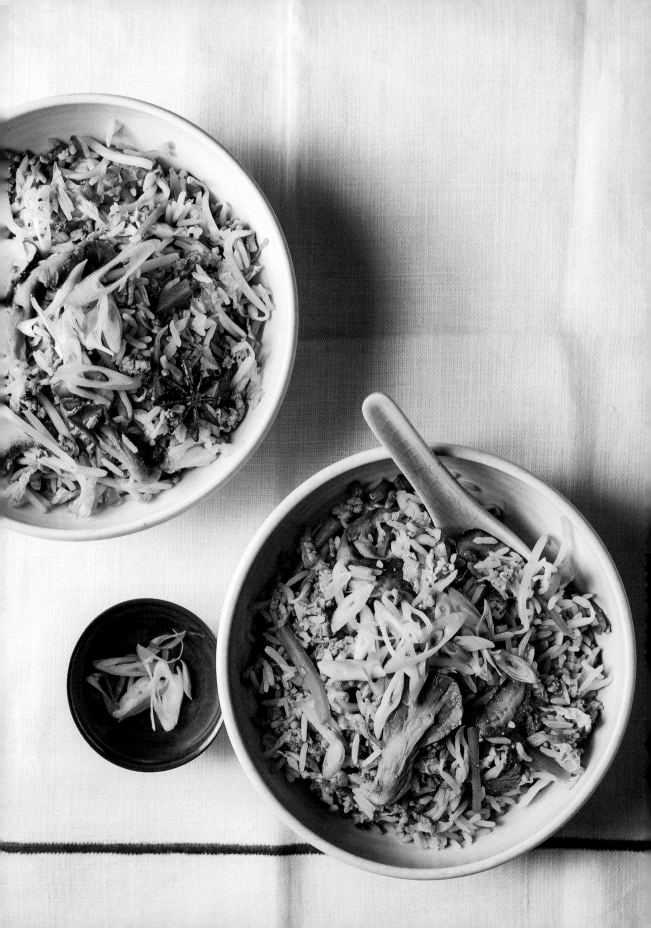

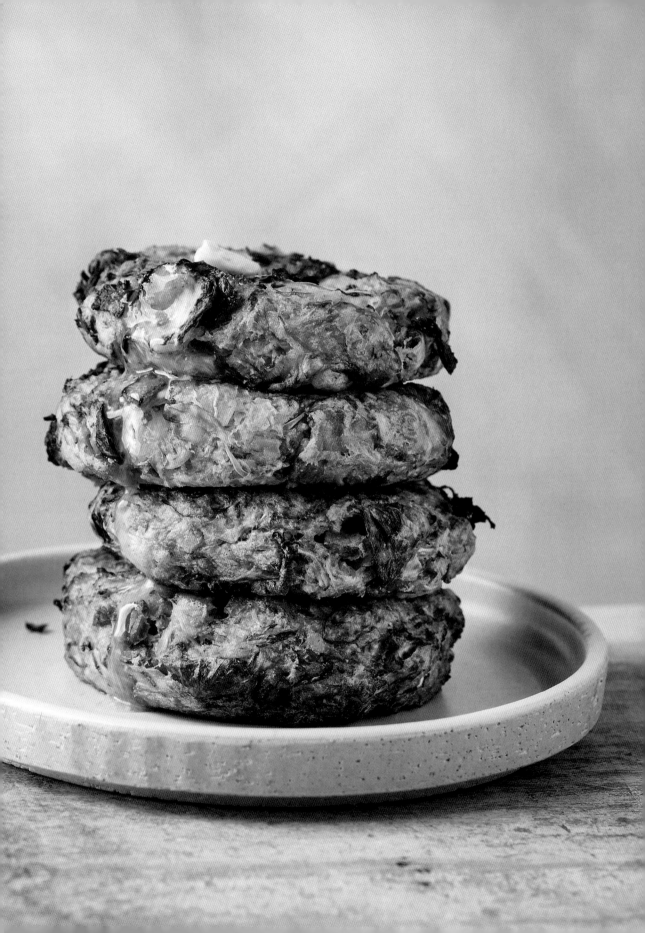

SERVES 4
PREP: **15 MINS**
COOK: **21 MINS**

HAM AND BRUSSELS SPROUTS BUBBLE AND SQUEAK CAKES

1 onion, finely diced

olive oil spray

455g (1lb) yellow-fleshed potatoes (skin on)

200g (7oz) Brussels sprouts, shredded (or use a mixture of Brussels sprouts and Savoy cabbage)

2 garlic cloves, crushed

½ tsp paprika

120ml (4fl oz) hot chicken stock

100g (3½oz) thick sliced ham, chopped

salt and freshly ground black pepper

1 tbsp melted butter

1. Preheat the air fryer to 190°C/375°F for 2 minutes.

2. Line the air fryer basket with non-stick baking paper and spray with olive oil spray. Add the onion with a pinch of salt and spray with olive oil spray. Air-fry for 5 minutes.

3. While the onion is cooking, microwave the potatoes for 6–8 minutes – they should be soft when gently squeezed. Set aside to cool slightly.

4. Once the onion has cooked for 5 minutes, add the Brussels sprouts, garlic, paprika and stock and mix to combine.

5. Air-fry for a further 6 minutes until the sprouts are softened and only a small amount of the stock remains.

6. Remove the skin from the potatoes and place in a bowl. Add the Brussels sprouts and onion mixture along with the cooked ham, and mix until well combined. Season to taste with salt and black pepper.

7. Spray your hands with olive oil spray and shape the mixture into 4 rough patties, compressing them well together. Add to the air fryer, brush one side with half the melted butter and air-fry for 5–6 minutes at 190°C/375°F, until lightly golden on top. Turn carefully, brush the other side with the remaining butter and cook for an additional 5–6 minutes until golden on the other side.

Tip
These are great as a side dish in place of regular potatoes or we love these served with baked beans and a fried egg.

KCALS per serving 192   FAT 5.3g   SAT FAT 2.5g   CARBS 24g   SUGARS 4g   FIBRE 5.3g   PROTEIN 9.4g   SALT 0.76g

500g (1lb 2oz) potatoes
  (skin on), diced
½ tsp salt
¼ tsp freshly ground
  black pepper
½ tsp sweet paprika
¾ tsp onion granules
¾ tsp garlic granules
olive oil spray
100g (3½oz) lean bacon,
  sliced into strips
1 green (bell) pepper,
  thinly sliced
1 small onion, thinly sliced
4 large eggs
5 tbsp reduced-fat
  green pesto
60g (2oz) Cheddar, grated

CHEDDAR PESTO EGGS WITH POTATOES AND BACON

1. Preheat the air fryer to 200°C/400°F for 2 minutes.

2. Mix the potato in a bowl with the salt, pepper, paprika, onion granules and garlic granules. Spray with olive oil spray and toss to coat.

3. When the air fryer is hot, place the coated potato cubes directly in the basket or use a foil/silicone liner that fits. Spray with olive oil spray and air-fry for 15 minutes. Toss a few times throughout cooking to ensure even browning and spray with olive oil spray one more time.

4. Add in the bacon, green (bell) pepper and onion and air-fry for 5 minutes, then stir.

5. Reduce the temperature to 190°C/375°F. Make 4 wells in the potato mixture and crack in the eggs. Spray the top of the eggs with olive oil spray and air-fry for 4 minutes.

6. Roughly spoon the pesto on top and a scatter over the Cheddar. Air-fry for a further 2 minutes until the eggs are cooked and the cheese is melted.

Side suggestions

Delicious as it is or served with some toast and avocado.

KCALS per serving 341   FAT 17.4g   SAT FAT 6.4g   CARBS 23.8g   SUGARS 3.2g   FIBRE 4.4g   PROTEIN 20.1g   SALT 1.97g

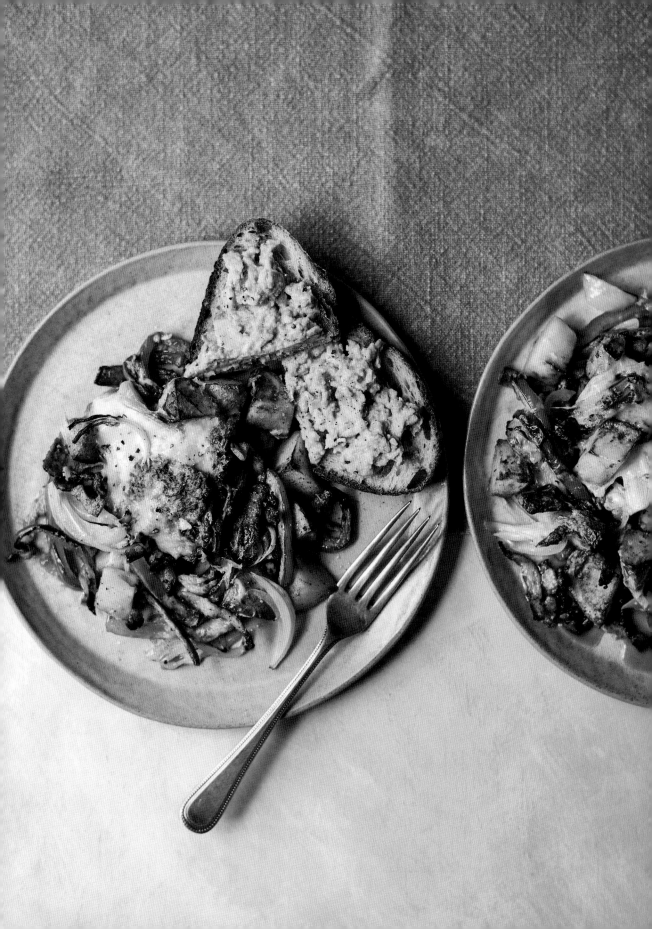

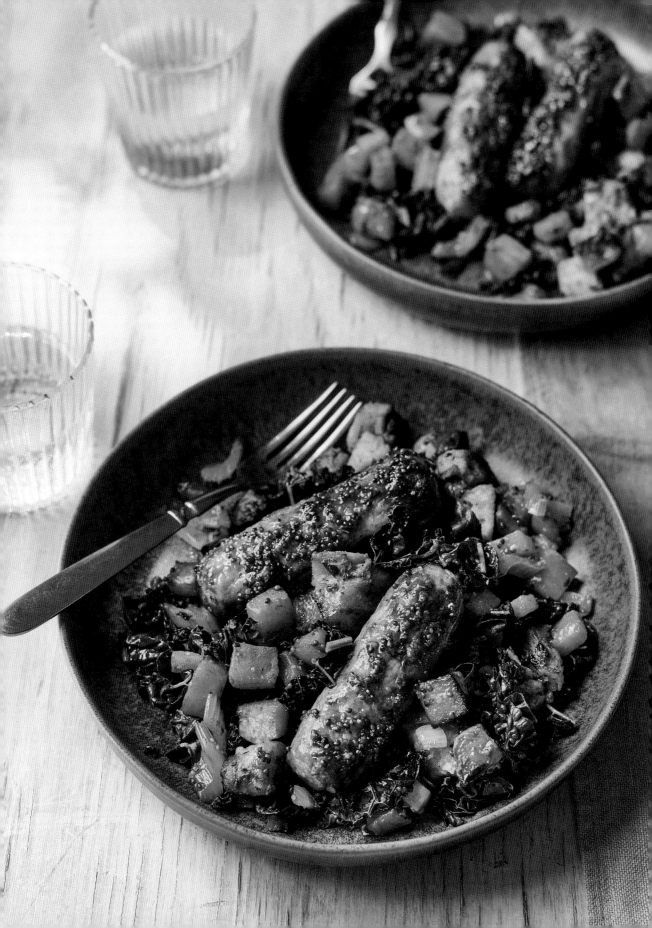

SERVES 4
PREP: **15 MINS**
COOK: **33 MINS**

HONEY AND MUSTARD SAUSAGES WITH BUTTERNUT SQUASH

2 tbsp honey

2 tbsp wholegrain mustard

455g (1lb) butternut
    squash, cubed

1 tsp sweet paprika

olive oil spray

60g (2oz) onion, chopped

60g (2oz) celery, chopped

2 tsp butter, melted

¼ tsp dried rosemary

¼ tsp dried sage

80g (2¾oz) bread, cut
    into cubes (see Tip)

120ml (4fl oz) hot
    chicken stock

8 reduced-fat sausages

250g (9oz) kale

2 garlic cloves, crushed

salt and freshly ground
    black pepper

Tip

*This recipe is best made
with bread that is at
least a day old. Use a
bakery loaf if possible.*

Swaps

*You can also swap the kale for
some shredded Savoy cabbage
or Brussels sprouts (you'll
need to blanch them first).*

1. Preheat the air fryer to 195°C/380°F for 2 minutes.

2. Mix the honey and mustard in a bowl and set aside.

3. Place the butternut squash directly into the air fryer basket (or use a foil/silicone liner that fits). Add the paprika with a pinch of salt, spray with olive oil and toss to coat. Air-fry for 5 minutes.

4. Push the butternut squash to one half of the air fryer basket. Toss the onion and celery in the melted butter with the rosemary and sage, season with salt and pepper and add to the other half of the basket.

5. Air-fry for a further 10–15 minutes until the butternut squash is tender. Turn the squash halfway through.

6. Remove the squash and set aside. Remove the onion and celery and add to a bowl with the bread cubes. Pour in the stock, a little at a time, until the bread is just moist (don't let it get soggy – you may not need it all). Mix to combine and season to taste.

7. Pierce the sausages with a fork and place them directly in the air fryer basket. Air-fry for 8 minutes until they are golden, turning them halfway through the cooking time, then remove (don't worry about them not being fully cooked at this stage).

9. Place the butternut squash back in the air fryer basket along with the kale. Add the garlic and toss to coat. Place the sausages on top, then scatter the stuffing mix in rough spoonfuls in the spaces in between the sausages. Spray over the top with olive oil.

10. Brush half of the honey and mustard mix over the top of the sausages and air-fry for 5 minutes. Carefully flip over the sausages, brush with remaining honey and mustard glaze and cook for a further 5 minutes, then serve.

KCALS per serving 345   FAT 10.1g   SAT FAT 3.4g   CARBS 38.1g   SUGARS 18.7g   FIBRE 10.2g   PROTEIN 20.5g   SALT 2.31g

SERVES 4
PREP: 10 MINS
COOK: 14 MINS

1 tbsp American
    yellow mustard

4 pork shoulder steaks
    (approx. 500g/17oz
    total weight), trimmed
    of visible fat

1½ tbsp sweet paprika

½ tsp onion granules

½ tsp garlic granules

¼ tsp salt

¼ tsp freshly ground
    black pepper

¼ tsp cayenne pepper
    (optional)

For the sauce

4 tbsp barbecue sauce

4 tbsp apple juice

60g (2oz) passata

SMOKED ST LOUIS BBQ PORK STEAKS

1. Rub the mustard into the pork steaks. Sprinkle over all the seasonings and turn until the pork is well coated.

2. Preheat the air fryer to 200°C/400°F for 2 minutes.

3. Place the pork steaks directly into the air fryer basket or use a foil/silicone liner that fits. Air-fry for 8 minutes until the pork is cooked, turning halfway through cooking.

4. To make the sauce, mix all the ingredients together in a bowl until well combined.

5. Brush half of the sauce over the top of the pork and air-fry for 3 minutes.

6. Turn the pork steaks again and brush the remaining sauce over the other side. Cook for a final 3 minutes.

Side suggestions

Any potato side dish with sweetcorn and/or green beans would make perfect accompaniments to this recipe.

KCALS per serving 203   FAT 7.8g   SAT FAT 2.6g   CARBS 7.7g   SUGARS 6.7g   FIBRE 1.8g   PROTEIN 24.6g   SALT 0.94g

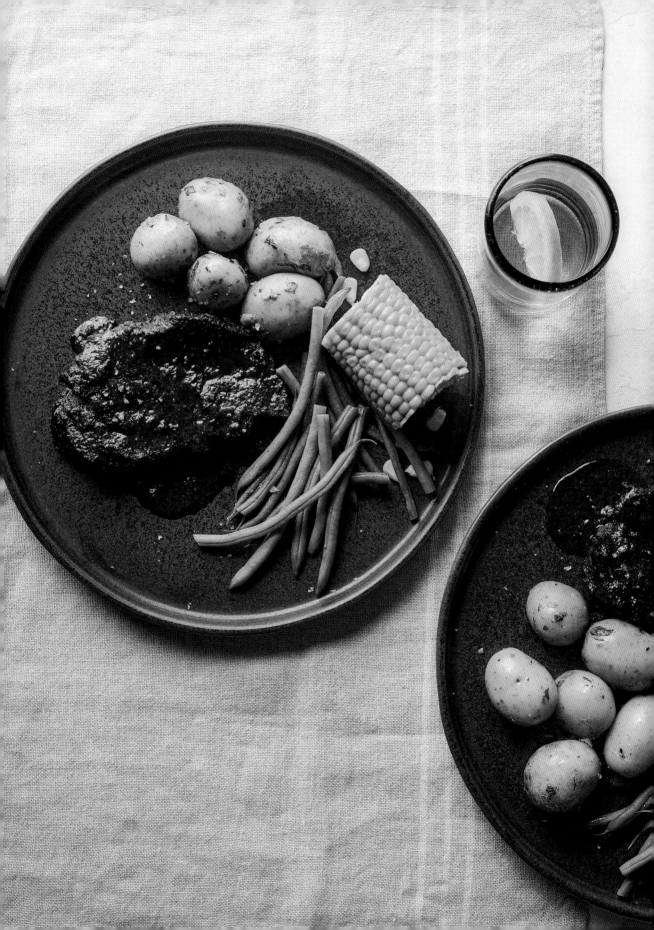

SAUSAGE AND GNOCCHI BAKE

4 reduced-fat pork sausages of choice (approx. 375g/13oz in weight), skin removed and meat broken into pieces

1 tsp sweet paprika

1 tsp herbes de Provence

1 onion, finely diced

olive oil spray

2 garlic cloves, crushed

500g (1lb 2oz) gnocchi

100g (3½oz) light cream cheese

240ml (8½fl oz) hot chicken stock

½ tsp red chilli flakes

30g (1oz) Parmesan, freshly grated

2 handfuls of spinach, stems removed

100g (3½oz) mozzarella, broken into pieces

1. Place the sausage meat in a bowl with the paprika and herbes de Provence. Add the onion and garlic and mix to combine. Spray with olive oil spray.

2. Preheat the air fryer to 190°C/375°F for 2 minutes.

3. Place the sausage mix directly into the air fryer basket in an even layer or use a foil/silicone liner that fits. Air-fry for 5 minutes until browned.

4. Stir the sausage, breaking up any large lumps, then add the gnocchi and mix to combine. Cook for a further 5 minutes.

5. Mix the cream cheese with the hot stock in a jug. Whisk until they are combined and the cream cheese is melted.

6. Add the creamy sauce to the sausages along with the chilli flakes and half the Parmesan and mix until combined.

7. Stir in the spinach until just wilted. Top with the mozzarella and remaining Parmesan and cook for a final 4–5 minutes until the cheese is just melted and lightly golden.

Side suggestions

For a filling meal, serve with some additional vegetables or a side salad.

KCALS per serving 477   FAT 14.1g   SAT FAT 7.4g   CARBS 55.3g   SUGARS 6.8g   FIBRE 6.9g   PROTEIN 28.8g   SALT 2.52g

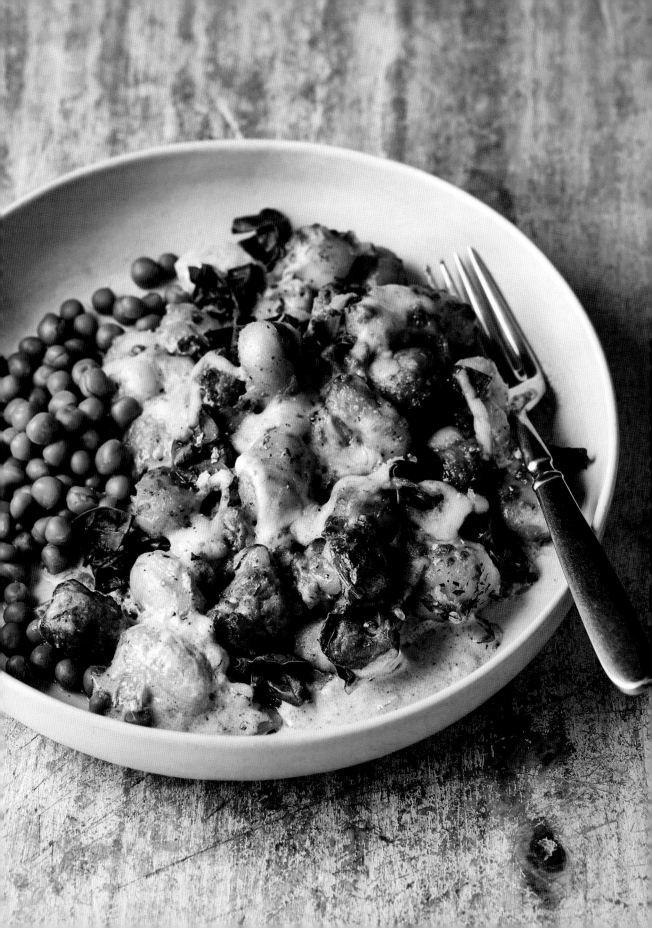

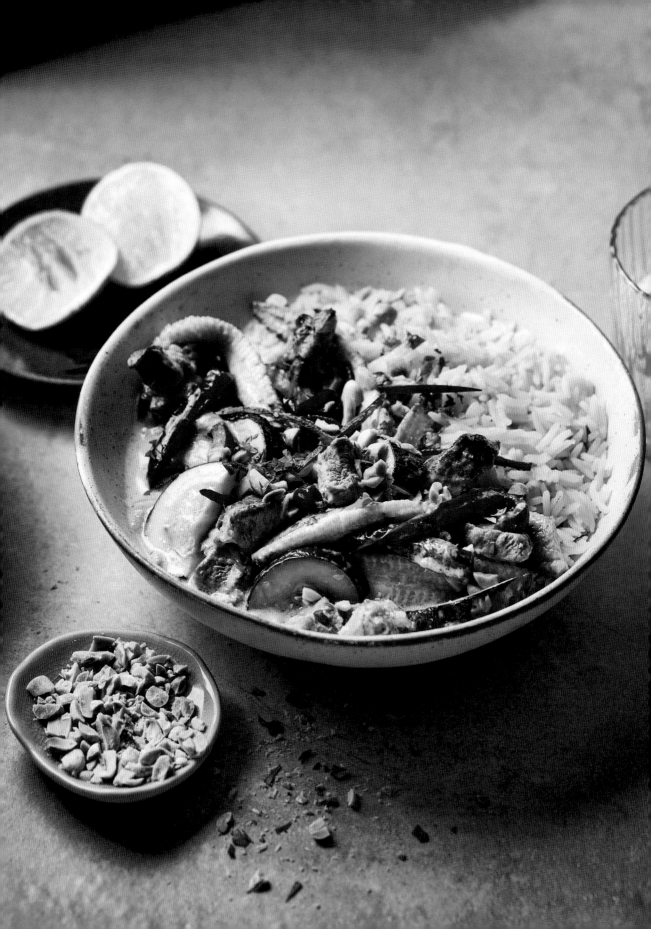

SERVES 4
PREP: **10 MINS**
COOK: **23 MINS**

THAI GREEN PORK CURRY

455g (1lb) pork shoulder
  steaks (trimmed of
  visible fat), sliced into
  bite-sized pieces

1 small onion, diced

2 garlic cloves, crushed

2 tsp grated fresh ginger

olive oil spray

2–3 tbsp Thai Green
  curry paste

400g (14oz) can light
  coconut milk

½ tbsp cornflour (cornstarch)

1 tbsp fish sauce

1 tbsp lemongrass paste

1 tbsp granulated sweetener

1 courgette (zucchini)
  (approx. 160g/5¾oz)

½ red (bell) pepper,
  thinly sliced

12 baby corn

squeeze of fresh lime juice

salt and freshly ground
  black pepper

To serve

lime wedges

handful of freshly chopped
  coriander (cilantro)

sliced red chillies

2 tbsp chopped peanuts
  (optional)

1. Preheat the air fryer to 200°C/400°F.

2. Place the pork directly into the air fryer basket or use a foil/silicone liner that fits. Add the onion, garlic, ginger and a little salt and pepper. Spray all over with olive oil spray.

3. Air-fry for 8 minutes until the pork is cooked, tossing halfway through.

4. Add the Thai curry paste with a splash of coconut milk and stir until well combined.

5. Mix the remaining coconut milk with the cornflour and pour this over the pork with the fish sauce. Add the lemongrass paste, sweetener, courgette, red (bell) pepper and baby corn. Air-fry for 15–17 minutes.

6. Squeeze in a little juice from a fresh lime and serve with additional lime wedges, chopped coriander, sliced red chilli and chopped peanuts, if you like.

Note

Use a good brand of Thai curry paste for the best taste.

KCALS per serving 300 FAT 16.5g SAT FAT 8.7g CARBS 11.7g SUGARS 4.6g FIBRE 2.8g PROTEIN 24.7g SALT 1.5g

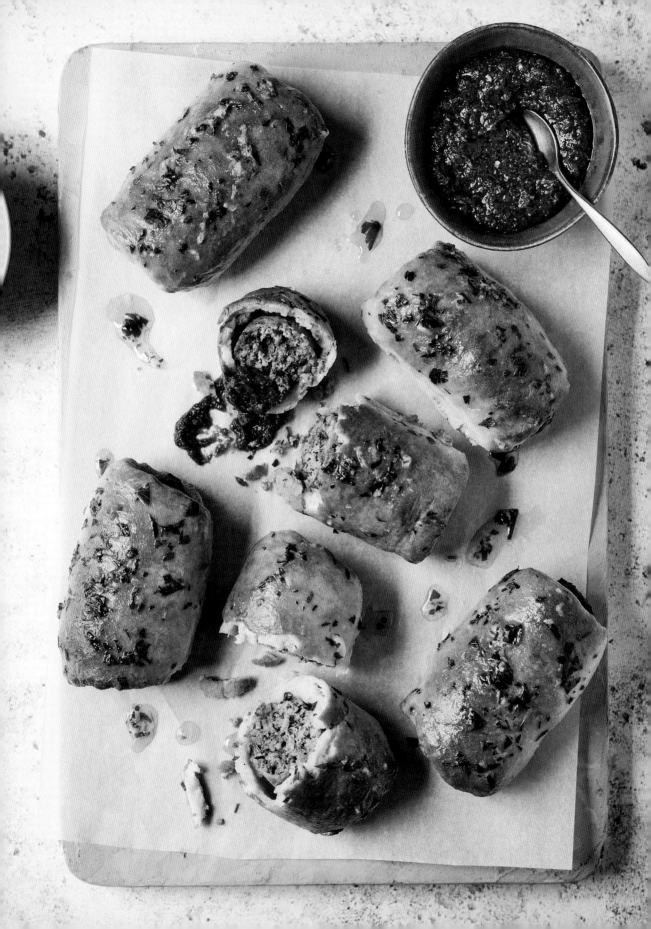

GARLIC BREAD SAUSAGE ROLLS WITH MARINARA SAUCE

500g (1lb 2oz) 5% fat pork mince (ground pork)

1 tbsp maple syrup

olive oil spray

160g (5¾oz) self-raising flour

180g (6½oz) fat-free Greek yogurt (see Tip)

1 tbsp butter, melted

2 garlic cloves, crushed

1 tbsp finely chopped fresh parsley

10g (¼oz) fresh Parmesan, finely grated

2 garlic cloves, minced

pinch of salt

For the marinara sauce

80g (6½oz) passata

1 tbsp tomato purée (paste)

1 tsp sugar or granulated sweetener

½ tsp garlic granules

½ tsp dried basil

½ tsp dried oregano

For the Italian seasoning mix

1 tsp sweet paprika

1 tsp dried parsley

½ tsp salt

½ tsp garlic granules

pinch of freshly ground black pepper

¼ tsp dried rosemary

¼ tsp fennel seeds, crushed

¼ tsp dried thyme

¼ tsp dried oregano

pinch of red chilli flakes (optional)

1. To make the marinara sauce, whisk the ingredients in a jug until well combined, then set aside.

2. To make the Italian seasoning, mix the ingredients together in a bowl.

3. Place the pork mince in a separate bowl and mix with the maple syrup and Italian seasoning mix. Grease your hands with olive oil spray and shape the mixture into 6 sausages.

4. Preheat the air fryer to 200°C/400°F for a couple of minutes.

5. Line the air fryer basket with non-stick baking paper and spray with olive oil spray. Add the sausages and air-fry for 5–6 minutes, until they are lightly golden and almost cooked through (it doesn't matter if they are still a little undercooked in the middle). Remove and set aside.

6. Place the flour and Greek yogurt in a bowl and mix with a wooden spoon or spatula until the mixture forms a ball. Roll the ball around the sides of the bowl to collect any additional flour/dough stuck to the edges.

7. Transfer the dough to a lightly floured surface and knead it a couple of times, then divide into 6 pieces and roll out each one into a rectangular shape that is roughly the same length as the sausage and just over double the width.

8. Place a sausage in the centre of one of the rectangles and fold the dough around the sausage to make a sausage roll (the ends should be open). Pinch the dough roughly to seal.

9. Place each sausage roll in the air fryer seam-side down and air-fry for 10 minutes at 180°C/350°F, turning for the last 3 minutes.

10. Mix the butter and garlic in a bowl with the fresh parsley. Brush over the top of the sausage rolls, sprinkle with Parmesan and serve with the marinara sauce on the side, warmed slightly if you prefer.

Tip

It's important to use Greek yogurt here, not Greek-style yogurt – otherwise you won't get a proper dough.

KCALS per serving 270 FAT 7.3g SAT FAT 3.3g CARBS 25.7g SUGARS 4.3g FIBRE 1.9g PROTEIN 24.4g SALT 1g

SERVES 4
PREP: 10 MINS
COOK: 15 MINS

4 pork shoulder steaks
  (approx. 500g/1lb 2oz),
  trimmed of visible fat
  and thinly sliced
1 tsp cornflour (cornstarch)
½ tsp bicarbonate of
  soda (baking soda)
40g (1½oz) brown sugar
1 tbsp fish sauce
1 tbsp light soy sauce
1 tsp dark soy sauce
pinch of red chilli flakes
½ tbsp lemongrass paste
olive oil spray
pinch of ground black pepper
½ small red onion, thinly sliced
2 garlic cloves, crushed
1 tsp grated fresh ginger

To serve
handful of finely chopped
  fresh coriander
2 spring onions
  (scallions), sliced
1 red chilli, sliced

CARAMELIZED VIETNAMESE PORK

1. Place the pork in a bowl. Add the cornflour and bicarbonate of soda with 1 tablespoon water and leave to soak for 15 minutes.

2. Mix the sugar, fish sauce, light and dark soy sauces, chilli flakes and lemongrass paste in a separate bowl and add 3 tablespoons water.

3. Preheat the air fryer to 200°C/400°F for 2 minutes.

4. Spray the pork with olive oil spray and place it directly in the air fryer basket or use a foil/silicone liner that fits. Add a pinch of black pepper and air-fry for 5–6 minutes until it is lightly browned/caramelized around the edges. Turn the pork pieces halfway through. Remove and set aside.

5. Place the onion, garlic and ginger in the air fryer basket. Spray with more olive oil spray and cook for 2 minutes.

6. Stir in the sauce and cook for a further 3 minutes, then add the pork and cook for 5 minutes.

7. To serve, scatter with coriander, spring onion and sliced red chilli.

Side suggestions
This is great served with white rice, cucumber slices and julienned carrot or, for a lighter meal, in crunchy lettuce wraps.

KCALS per serving 222 FAT 7.7g SAT FAT 2.5g CARBS 13.5g SUGARS 11.5g FIBRE 0.5g PROTEIN 24.2g SALT 2.26g

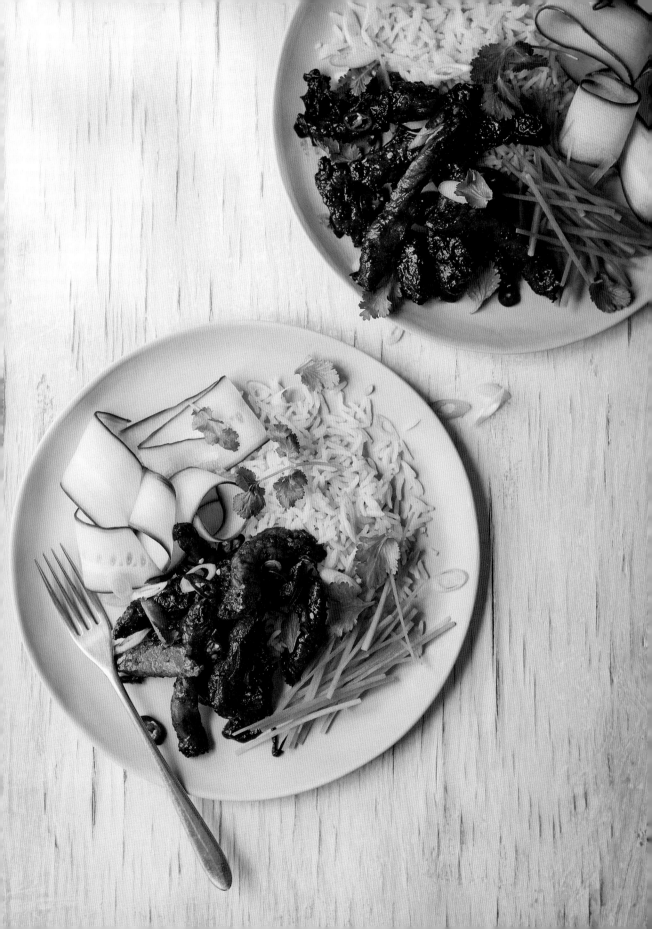

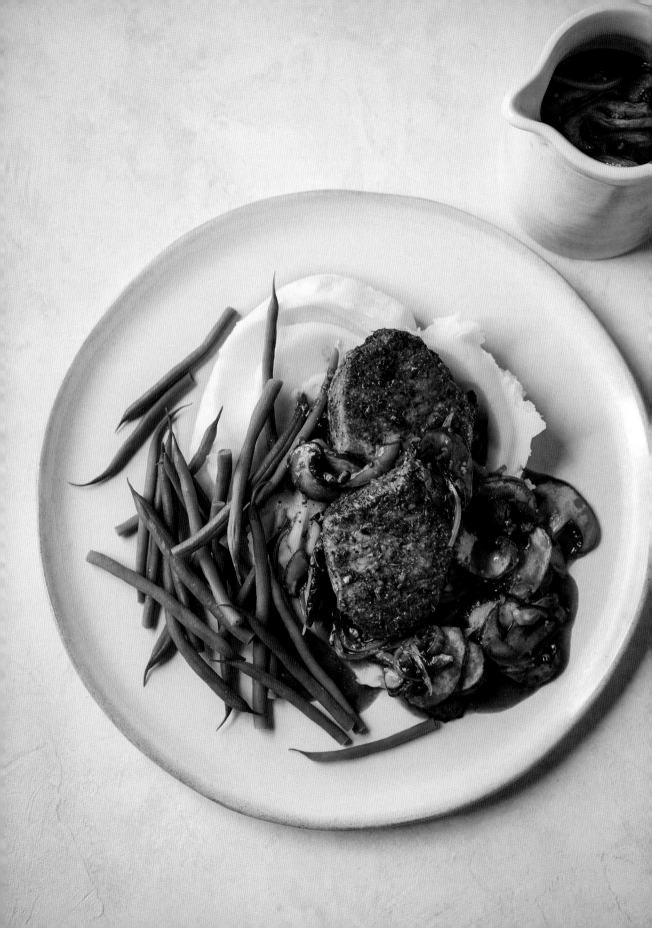

PORK WITH RICH MUSHROOM AND ONION GRAVY

4 pork shoulder steaks
  (approx. 500g/1lb 2oz),
  halved and trimmed of fat

1 tsp sweet paprika

1 tsp herbes de Provence

½ tsp garlic granules

½ tsp onion granules

½ tsp salt

¼ tsp freshly ground
  black pepper

200g (7oz) mushrooms,
  thinly sliced

1 onion, halved and
  thinly sliced

2 garlic cloves, crushed

olive oil spray

240ml (8½fl oz) hot
  chicken stock

1 tbsp tomato purée (paste)

1 tbsp balsamic vinegar

½ tbsp dark soy sauce

1 tsp wholegrain mustard

1 tbsp cornflour (cornstarch)

salt and freshly ground
  black pepper

fresh thyme or parsley
  leaves, to garnish

1. Preheat the air fryer to 200°C/400°F for 2 minutes.

2. Place the pork in a bowl and add the paprika, herbes de Provence, garlic granules, onion granules and salt and black pepper.

3. Place the mushrooms, onion and garlic directly in the air fryer basket or use a foil/silicone liner that fits. Top with the seasoned pork shoulder steaks, spray over the top with olive oil spray and air-fry for 5 minutes, then turn the pork and cook for a further 4–5 minutes until browned on both sides. Remove and set aside.

4. Whisk the hot stock in a jug with the tomato purée, balsamic vinegar, soy sauce and wholegrain mustard.

5. Mix the cornflour with a little water to make a slurry, then add this to the stock and whisk again to combine.

6. Stir the stock into the mushroom mixture and air-fry for 5 minutes until it thickens slightly, then add the pork back in and air-fry for a further 3 minutes.

7. Adjust the seasoning if necessary and serve garnished with fresh thyme leaves or parsley.

Side suggestions
Mashed potato or cauliflower with some greens of your choice would be perfect here.

KCALS per serving 220 FAT 8g SAT FAT 2.6g CARBS 8.7g SUGARS 3.9g FIBRE 2.2g PROTEIN 27.3g SALT 1.51g

BACON, CHEDDAR AND SWEETCORN FRITTERS

3 slices of smoked
  lean back bacon, fat
  removed, finely diced
olive oil spray
400g (14oz) can
  sweetcorn, drained
50g (1¾oz) plain
  (all-purpose) flour
½ tbsp cornflour (cornstarch)
50g Cheddar, grated
1 egg
2 tbsp plain fat-free
  Greek yogurt
2 spring onions (scallions),
  green part only, sliced
½ tsp garlic granules
pinch of red chilli
  flakes (optional)
pinch of salt and freshly
  ground black pepper

1. Preheat the air fryer to 190°C/380°F for 2 minutes.

2. Add the bacon directly to the air fryer basket or use a foil/silicone liner that fits. Spray with olive oil and air-fry for about 6 minutes until golden brown. Remove and set aside.

3. Mix the sweetcorn, flour, cornflour, Cheddar, egg, yogurt, spring onions, garlic granules, chilli flakes (if using) and salt and pepper in a bowl. Add in the cooked bacon and toss to combine.

4. Line the air fryer basket with non-stick baking paper and spray with olive oil spray. I recommend cooking the fritters in two batches. Add equal-sized dollops of the mixture (approximately 2 heaped tablespoons per fritter) to the air fryer basket and flatten slightly (this should make about 8 fritters). Don't place them too close together or they will be hard to flip.

5. Air-fry the fritters for 8–10 minutes until golden and cooked through, flipping halfway through.

Side suggestions

Serve the fritters with soured cream, lettuce, diced cherry tomatoes or salsa and avocado. They are also delicious topped with an egg.

Extras

Make a tasty dip by mixing 2 tbsp light mayonnaise with 2 tbsp sweet chilli sauce.

Vegetarian

For a vegetarian version, omit the bacon.

KCALS per serving 267   FAT 11.7g   SAT FAT 4.9g   CARBS 23.8g   SUGARS 7.1g   FIBRE 3.2g   PROTEIN 15g   SALT 0.96g

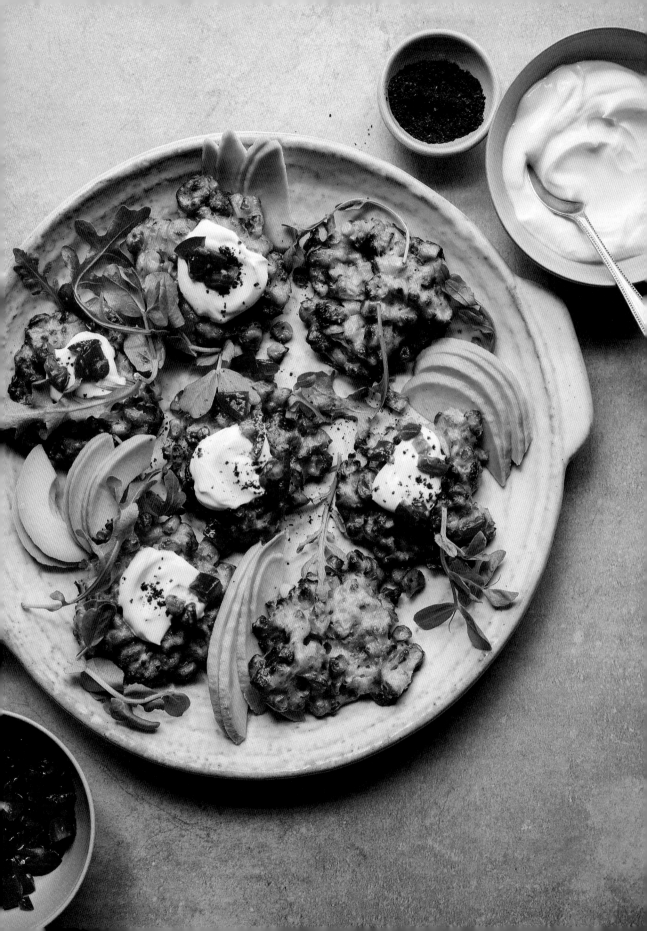

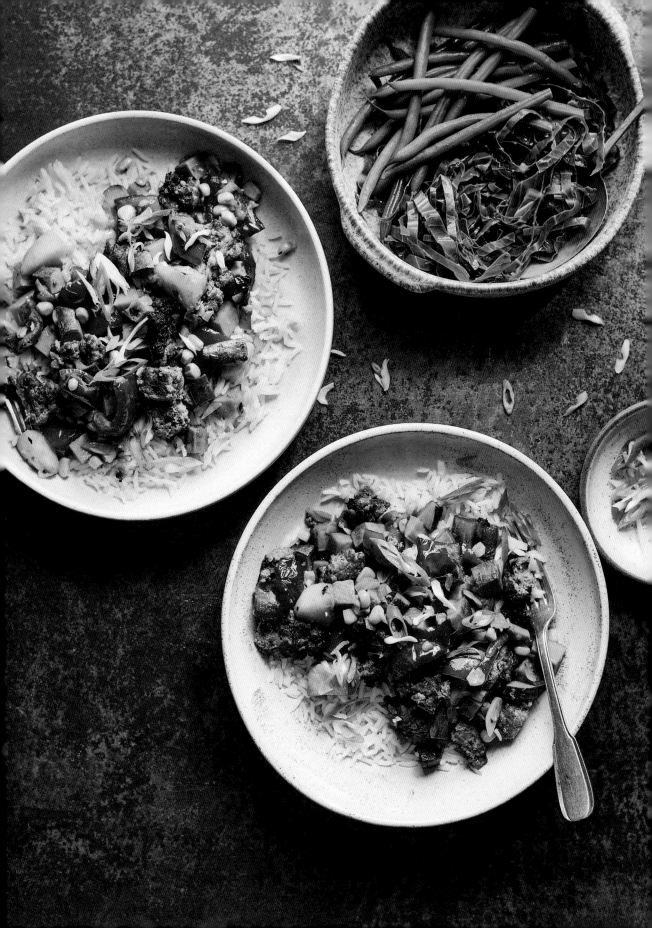

SERVES 4
PREP: **10 MINS**
COOK: **26 MINS**

455g (1lb) 5% fat pork
   mince (ground pork)
1 tbsp honey
300g (10½oz) sweet potato,
   peeled and finely cubed
150g (5½oz) onion, diced
3 garlic cloves, crushed
1 apple, peeled and diced
1 red (bell) pepper, diced
1 green (bell) pepper, diced
olive oil spray
85g (3oz) canned or
   frozen sweetcorn
120ml (4fl oz) hot
   chicken stock
salt and freshly ground
   black pepper
chopped spring onions
   (scallions), to serve

For the seasoning
1 tbsp sweet paprika
1 tsp garlic granules
1 tsp onion granules
½ tsp dried oregano
½ tsp cayenne pepper
pinch of dried thyme

CAJUN PORK WITH SWEET POTATO AND APPLE

1. To make the seasoning, mix the ingredients together in a bowl until well combined.

2. Place the pork mince in a bowl. Reserve a teaspoon of the seasoning and add the rest to the pork with a pinch of salt and pepper. Add the honey and mix to combine.

3. Preheat the air fryer to 190°C/375°F for 2 minutes.

4. Place the pork directly into the air fryer basket (or use a foil/silicone liner that fits) and air-fry for 6 minutes until browned and lightly caramelized around the edges. Toss the mixture halfway through. Remove and set aside.

5. Place the sweet potato with the remaining seasoning in the air fryer, along with the onion, garlic, apple and red and green (bell) peppers. Season with salt and pepper and spray with olive oil. Air-fry for 12–15 minutes, tossing every 4–5 minutes, until the sweet potato is tender. Spray with more olive oil if necessary.

6. Add the pork back in along with the sweetcorn and hot stock, and increase the temperature to 200°C/400°F. Air-fry for a final 5 minutes, then sprinkle with chopped spring onion and serve.

Side suggestions
This is delicious just as it is but, for additional sides, serve with rice and some seasonal greens.

KCALS per serving 308   FAT 6.7g   SAT FAT 2.3g   CARBS 31.1g   SUGARS 15.3g   FIBRE 6.9g   PROTEIN 27.4g   SALT 0.44g

CUMIN-ROASTED PORK STEAKS WITH GARLIC GREEN BEANS

olive oil spray
4 pork shoulder steaks
   (500g/17oz each)
3 tbsp light mayonnaise
2 tsp curry powder
1½ tsp sweet paprika
2 tsp cumin seeds
pinch of red chilli flakes
1 tsp garlic granules
1 tbsp honey
½ tsp salt
¼ tsp freshly ground
   black pepper
lemon wedges, to serve

For the green beans
400g (14oz) green
   beans, trimmed
½ tsp garlic granules
½ tsp onion granules
salt and freshly ground
   black pepper
olive oil spray

1. To prepare the green beans, place them in a bowl with all the seasonings. Toss to coat and spray well with olive oil.

2. Preheat the air fryer to 190°C/375°F for 2 minutes.

3. Line the air fryer basket with non-stick baking paper and spray with olive oil spray. Add the green beans and cook for about 8 minutes until tender and slightly crisp. Remove and set aside.

4. Place the pork in a bowl and mix with the mayonnaise, curry powder, paprika, cumin seeds, chilli flakes, garlic granules and honey until evenly coated. Season both sides with the salt and black pepper.

5. Preheat the air fryer to 200°C/400°F for 2 minutes.

6. Add the pork steaks and spray over the top with olive oil. Air-fry for 8–9 minutes until cooked through, turning halfway through and spraying again with olive oil.

7. Transfer the pork steaks to a plate and rest for a few minutes. Add the green beans back to the air fryer basket and cook for a further minute just to warm through.

8. Serve with fresh lemon wedges and enjoy!

KCALS per serving 327   FAT 20.4g   SAT FAT 5.9g   CARBS 8.7g   SUGARS 6.4g   FIBRE 4.7g   PROTEIN 24.8g   SALT 0.83g

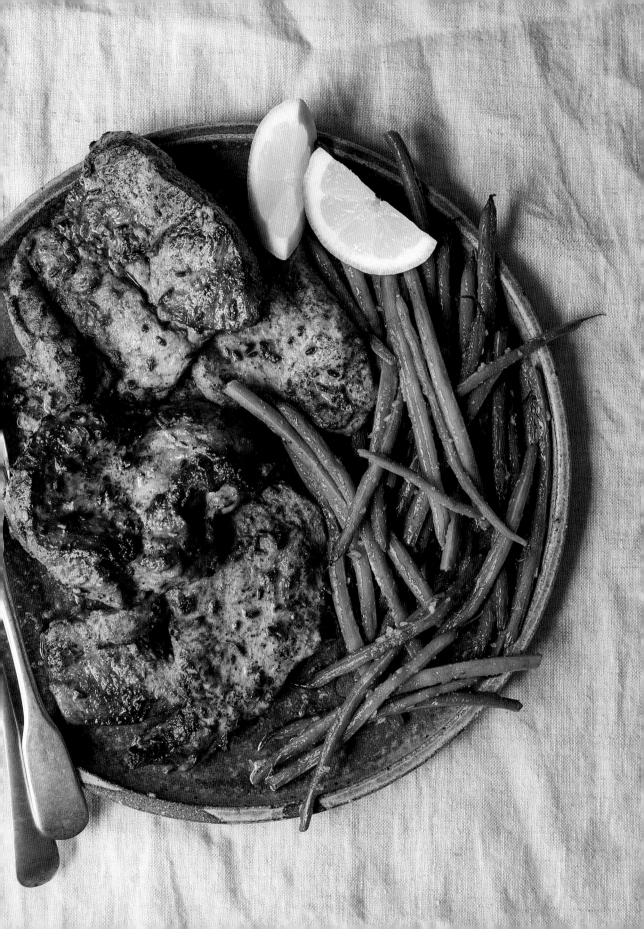

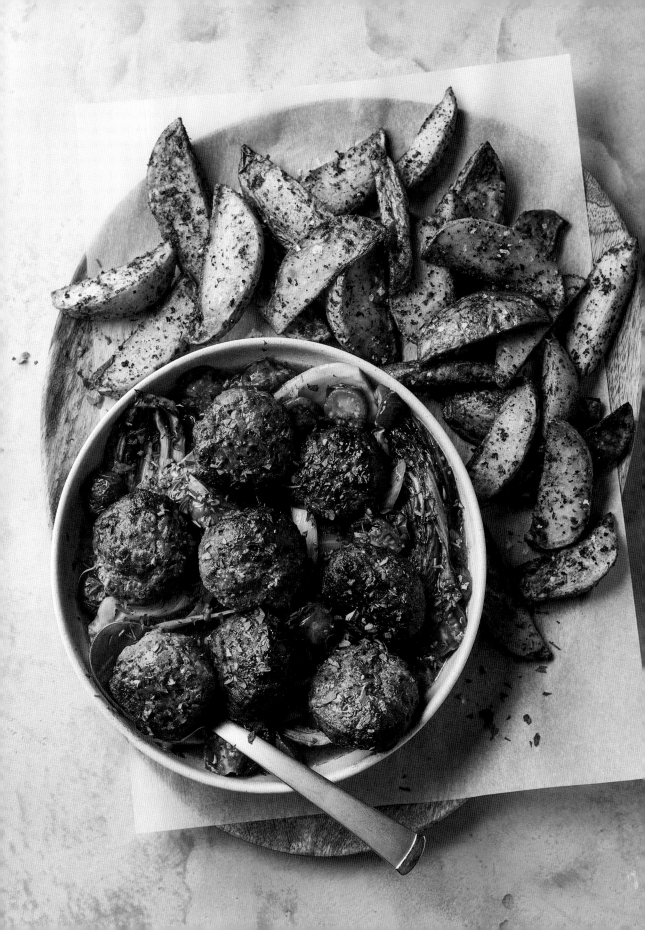

SERVES 4
PREP: **10 MINS**
COOK: **45 MINS**

400g (14oz) 5% fat pork
  mince (ground pork)
¼ tsp bicarbonate of
  soda (baking soda)
50g (1¾oz) Parmesan,
  freshly grated
50g (1¾oz) 'nduja paste
1 fennel bulb (250g/9oz),
  thinly sliced
olive oil spray
250g (9oz) baby plum
  tomatoes or cherry
  tomatoes, halved
3 garlic cloves, crushed
pinch of dried oregano
150ml (5fl oz) hot
  chicken stock
salt and freshly ground
  black pepper

**For the seasoned
potato wedges**
550g (1lb 2oz) potatoes,
  sliced into wedges
olive oil spray
1 tsp paprika
1 tsp dried parsley
¾ tsp garlic granules
¾ tsp onion granules
¾ tsp sea salt
½ tsp dried basil
½ tsp freshly ground
  black pepper
finely chopped fresh
  parsley or coriander
  (cilantro), to serve

MINI 'NDUJA PORK BURGERS WITH FENNEL, TOMATOES AND SEASONED POTATO WEDGES

1. To prepare the potato wedges, place them in a bowl and cover with water. Drop in some ice cubes and leave to soak for at least 30 minutes.

2. Drain the potatoes and pat dry with clean paper towels. Place in a bowl and spray with olive oil. Add all the seasonings and toss to coat.

3. Preheat the air fryer to 200°C/400°F for 2 minutes.

4. Line the air fryer basket with non-stick baking paper and spray with olive oil spray. Add the wedges, spray over the top with more olive oil and air-fry for 20 minutes until golden. Turn the potatoes halfway through cooking and spray again with olive oil. When cooked, remove and set aside.

5. Meanwhile, place the pork mince in a bowl and mix with the bicarbonate of soda, Parmesan, 'nduja paste and 2 tablespoons water. Spray your hands with olive oil spray and shape the mixture into 8 mini burger patties, then set aside.

6. Place the fennel in the air fryer basket (make sure to line it if your basket isn't solid) and add the tomatoes, garlic, oregano and stock with a pinch of salt and pepper. Toss to coat, spray over the top with olive oil spray and air-fry at 190°C/375°F for 13 minutes, stirring halfway through the cooking time.

7. Season both sides of the burger patties, then arrange them on top of the tomatoes and fennel. Spray over the top with olive oil spray and air-fry for 10–12 minutes until the burgers are cooked through. Turn the burgers halfway through cooking and spray with more olive oil spray.

8. Transfer the burgers with the tomato and fennel mixture to a plate. Return the potato wedges to the air fryer for a couple of minutes to reheat. (Don't worry if there are juices from the burgers in the air fryer – this is all amazing flavour from the 'nduja.)

9. Serve sprinkled with chopped parsley or coriander.

KCALS per serving 395   FAT 16.5g   SAT FAT 6.6g   CARBS 27.3g   SUGARS 6g   FIBRE 6.5g   PROTEIN 31g   SALT 2.28g

DETROIT-STYLE SUPREME PIZZA

110g (4oz) self-raising flour, plus extra for dusting

125g (4½oz) fat-free Greek yogurt

12 (25g) pepperoni slices

2 tbsp sliced black olives

¼ green (bell) pepper, thinly sliced

¼ red onion, thinly sliced

1–2 mushrooms, thinly sliced

50g (1¾oz) mozzarella, grated

30g (1oz) Cheddar, grated

For the sauce

100g (3½oz) passata

2½ tbsp tomato purée (paste)

½ tsp garlic granules

½ tsp onion granules

½ tsp dried basil

½ tsp dried oregano

1 tsp maple syrup

1. Place the flour and Greek yogurt in a bowl and combine with a wooden spoon or spatula until it forms a ball. Roll the ball around the sides of the bowl to collect any additional flour/dough that has stuck to the edges.

2. Place the dough ball on a lightly floured surface and knead a couple of times to ensure it is well mixed together. Roll out into a rough square 20cm x 20cm (8in. x 8 in.). (The Detroit-style pizza is traditionally a rectangle, but you can do it in a square to fit the air fryer.)

3. Preheat the air fryer to 180°C/350°F for 2 minutes.

4. Line the air fryer basket with non-stick baking paper and spray with olive oil. Add the pizza base and air-fry for 6 minutes. Turn the base for the last 2 minutes of cooking and remove the baking paper.

5. Add the pepperoni slices in vertical rows so they almost cover the base, then scatter over the olives, green (bell) pepper, mushroom and red onion.

6. Sprinkle over the mozzarella and Cheddar, making sure they reach the edge of the dough.

7. To make the sauce, mix the ingredients in a bowl until well combined. Drizzle 3 lines of sauce across the pizza base (this layering method is the hallmark of the Detroit-style pizza). Air-fry for 6–8 minutes until the cheese is golden and melted.

8. Slice the pizza in half down the middle vertically and then divide each half into 4 rectangular slices so that you have 8 in total. Serve with a mixed salad, if you like, and enjoy!

Tip

Want to serve 4? Simply double up the ingredients, make 2 pizzas and cook individually, following the method above. My kids have this pizza regularly and love it.

KCALS per serving 494   FAT 18g   SAT FAT 8.9g   CARBS 54.3g   SUGARS 11.5g   FIBRE 5.5g   PROTEIN 25.9g   SALT 1.97g

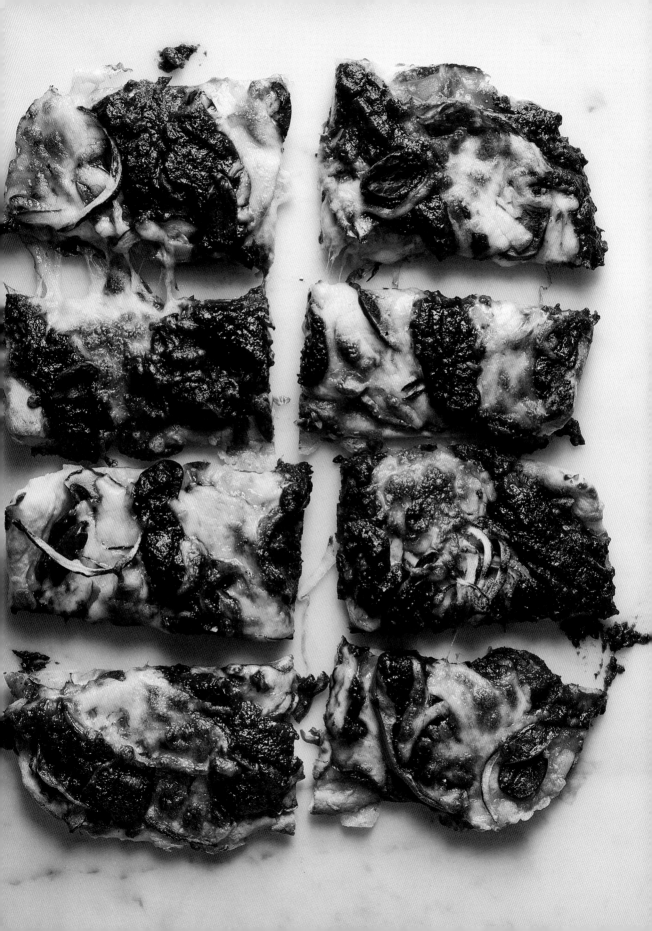

BEEF AND LAMB

PERI PERI STEAK WITH RICE 100

CREAMY COURGETTE-STUFFED
PASTA WITH BEEF AND PESTO 103

KOREAN-STYLE CORN DOGS 104

RENDANG-STYLE BEEF CURRY
WITH POTATOES 107

MONGOLIAN BEEF MEATBALLS 108

GREEK LAMB WITH ORZO 111

BEEF, CHORIZO AND
SUN-DRIED TOMATO RAGÙ
WITH PAPPARDELLE 112

RAS EL HANOUT LAMB
CHOPS WITH SWEET POTATO
AND CHICKPEAS 115

PEANUT BUTTER AND JALAPEÑO
RASPBERRY JAM BURGERS 116

CHILLI COFFEE STEAK
WITH RICE 119

BEEF NOODLE STIR-FRY 120

SEASONED STEAK WITH
CHIMICHURRI SAUCE AND
GARLIC WEDGES 123

FIRE MEATBALLS WITH
CHEESE 124

CHIPOTLE BEEF MACARONI 127

MONTREAL STEAK
BITE SKEWERS 128

THE ULTIMATE CHEESEBURGER
CHIMICHANGAS 130

PERSIAN-STYLE LAMB
HOTPOT 132

600g (1lb 5oz) sirloin
  steak (or any steak
  of your preference),
  trimmed of visible flat

coarse sea salt

For the steak marinade

1 tbsp sweet paprika

½ tsp smoked paprika

125g (4½oz) roasted
  red peppers in brine,
  well drained

1 tsp red chilli flakes
  (add more or less
  according to taste)

4 garlic cloves, crushed

¾ tsp dried oregano

1 tbsp finely chopped
  fresh basil

1 tbsp finely chopped
  fresh parsley

big handful of finely chopped
  fresh coriander (cilantro)

juice of ½ lemon

1½ tbsp honey

salt, to taste

For the rice

1 small onion, finely diced

½ red (bell) pepper,
  finely diced

½ green (bell) pepper
  finely diced

180g (6½oz) basmati rice

1 tbsp sweet paprika

1 tsp ground turmeric

¾ tsp ground cumin

1 tbsp tomato purée (paste)

salt and freshly ground
  black pepper

PERI PERI STEAK WITH RICE

1. To make the steak marinade, blitz all the ingredients in a mini food processor until you have a smooth paste.

2. Reserve 3 tablespoons of the marinade and set aside. Place the steak in a dish, add the remaining marinade and toss to coat, then place in the fridge to marinate overnight.

3. To make the peri peri mayo, whisk the reserved steak marinade with the Greek yogurt and light mayonnaise in a bowl and set aside.

4. Remove the steak from the fridge at least 20 minutes prior to cooking.

5. To make the rice, preheat a 20cm (8in.) cake barrel in the air fryer to 200°C/400°F for 2 minutes. Add the onion and (bell) peppers and air-fry for 5 minutes.

6. Add in the rice, paprika, turmeric, cumin, tomato pureé and a pinch of salt and black pepper, spray with olive oil and toss to coat.

7. Pour in the stock, cover tightly with foil and air-fry for 25 minutes. Remove the cake barrel from the air fryer and stir in the peas and sweetcorn. Wrap the barrel back up tightly with the foil and set aside while you cook the steak.

8. Preheat the air fryer again to 200°C/400°F for 2 minutes – just to ensure it is hot before adding the steak.

9. Remove the steak from the marinade, and season both sides with some coarse sea salt. Using the grill pan insert, add the steak to the air fryer basket, spray with olive oil and air-fry for 8–10 minutes (depending on thickness). Turn the steak halfway through cooking and spray the other side with oil. (Cook the steak for slightly longer if you like it more done.)

10. Let the steak rest for 8 minutes, then serve it sliced along with the rice, spicy peri peri mayo and sides of your choice.

KCALS per serving 542   FAT 12.9g   SAT FAT 3.8g   CARBS 53.5g   SUGARS 13.8g   FIBRE 6.2g   PROTEIN 49.9g   SALT 0.72g

olive oil spray

450ml (15fl oz) hot
  beef stock

40g (1½oz) frozen peas

40g (1½oz) frozen sweetcorn

For the creamy peri
  peri mayo

5 tbsp fat-free Greek yogurt

3 tbsp light mayonnaise

Side suggestions

Serve with a side salad (we love shredded crisp lettuce, red onion, tomato, cucumber) with the peri peri mayo. Avocado or grilled halloumi are also delicious for additional extras.

Swaps

Don't like the taste of coriander? Use a double portion of parsley for the marinade instead.

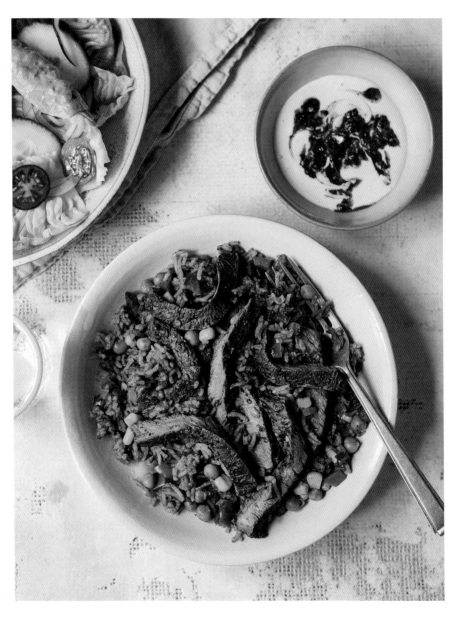

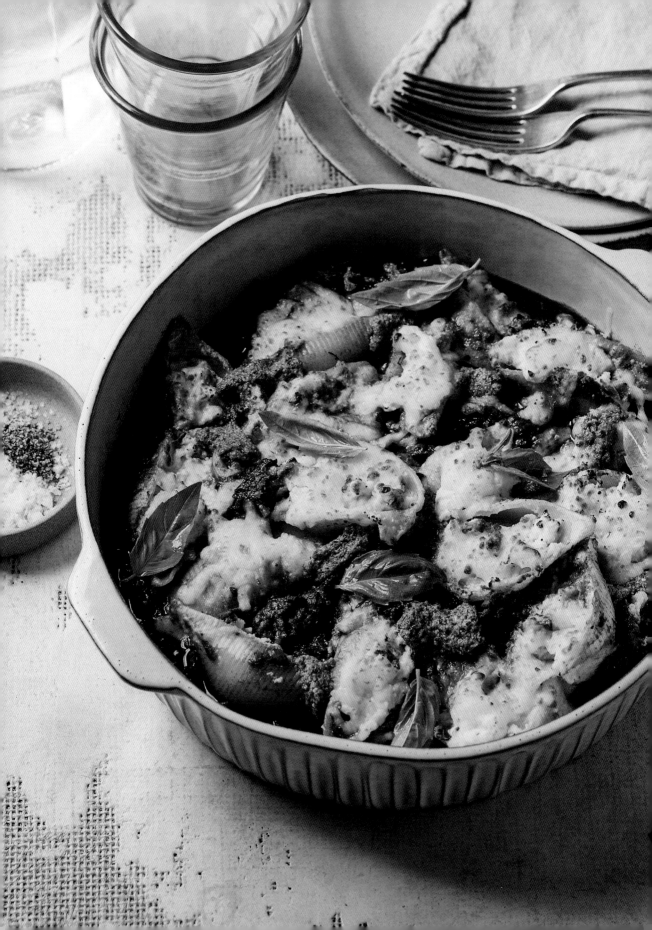

SERVES 4
PREP: **20 MINS**
COOK: **36 MINS**

CREAMY COURGETTE-STUFFED PASTA WITH BEEF AND PESTO

300g (10½oz) extra lean
  beef mince (ground beef)
1 onion, finely chopped
3 garlic cloves, crushed
1 tbsp sweet paprika
2 tsp dried parsley
1 tsp dried oregano
400g (14oz) can
  plum tomatoes
3 tbsp tomato purée (paste)
2 tsp sugar or sweetener
200ml (7fl oz) hot beef stock
20 jumbo dried pasta shells
100g (3½oz) courgettes
  (zucchini), finely
  grated and squeezed
  of excess moisture
270g (9½oz) ricotta
1 large egg
½ tsp garlic granules
½ tsp onion granules
30g (1oz) Parmesan,
  freshly grated
50g (1oz) mozzarella,
  freshly grated
4 tbsp reduced-fat
  green pesto
salt and ground black pepper
fresh basil leaves, to serve

1. Place the beef in a bowl with the onion, garlic, paprika, parsley, oregano and a pinch of salt and black pepper. Mix together until well combined.

2. Add a 20cm (8in.) cake barrel to the air fryer and preheat to 190°C/375°F for 2 minutes.

3. Place the beef mixture in the cake barrel and air-fry for 6 minutes. Roughly break up the meat halfway through cooking.

4. While the beef is cooking, crush the plum tomatoes in a jug, then add the tomato purée, sugar and hot stock and whisk to combine.

5. Pour the tomato mixture over the beef and air-fry for a further 15 minutes. Meanwhile, cook the pasta shells according to the packet instructions until al dente. Drain and set aside.

6. Pat the courgette dry with some paper towel and place in a bowl. Add the ricotta, egg, garlic and onion granules, a pinch of salt and black pepper and half the grated Parmesan. Mix until well combined.

7. Place about three-quarters of the meat mixture into a foil tray measuring approx. 20cm x 20cm (8in. x 8in.).

8. Fill the pasta shells with the courgette ricotta mixture and arrange these, evenly spaced out, on top of the meat sauce. Spoon the remaining meat sauce in between the shells to fill any gaps. Sprinkle the remaining Parmesan over the top along with the mozzarella.

9. Cover tightly with foil and air-fry at 180°C/350°F for 15 minutes, removing the foil for the final 5 minutes. Add the pesto randomly in half tablespoons on top for the last minute of cooking.

10. Serve scattered with fresh basil leaves.

Tip
If your air fryer has a solid basket, you can add the mixture directly to the air fryer in step 8.

KCALS per serving 512   FAT 21.2g   SAT FAT 10.6g   CARBS 38.5g   SUGARS 10.3g   FIBRE 6.2g   PROTEIN 38.6g   SALT 0.9g

KOREAN-STYLE CORN DOGS

4 beef hot dogs
160g (5¾oz) block of mozzarella (not in water, see Tip)
60g (2oz) cornflakes
1 tsp sweet paprika
½ tsp onion granules
½ tsp garlic granules
salt and freshly ground black pepper
2 tbsp cornflour (cornstarch)
2 medium eggs
olive oil spray

Side suggestions

Light mayonnaise, ketchup, sweet chilli, barbecue, sriracha sauce and mustard in any combination.

Swaps

Use pork or chicken hot dogs instead of the beef, if you prefer.

Tip

If you can't find a block of mozzarella, use mild Cheddar instead.

1. Slice each hot dog in half widthways, then cut the cheese to measure roughly the same as the hot dog halves – you should have 8 pieces of hot dog and 8 pieces of cheese – each piece of cheese should weigh about 20g (¾oz).

2. Place the cheese on a tray and freeze for 20 minutes to firm up.

3. Crush the cornflakes into fine crumbs in a bag. Add the paprika, onion and garlic granules with a pinch of salt and pepper and mix to combine.

4. Add half a hot dog and one piece of the cheese to a skewer. Repeat with the remaining hot dogs and cheese slices so that you have 8 skewers in total (make sure the skewers aren't too big as they will need to fit in the air fryer).

5. Pace the skewers on a plate and sprinkle over 1 tablespoon of the cornflour, ensuring they are well covered. Turn the skewers and add the other tablespoon of cornflour.

6. Sprinkle the crushed cornflakes onto a board and spread out in an even layer.

7. Whisk the eggs in a wide, shallow dish – this must be big enough to dip the hot dogs in.

8. Dip one cornflour-dusted corn dog into the egg mixture and then roll it in the cornflakes until it is well covered. If the cornflakes are not sticking well in some areas, just spray with a little oil and sprinkle with cornflakes – the cheese part must be fully covered. Repeat with the other corn dogs.

9. Preheat the air fryer to 170°C/350°F for 2 minutes.

10. Line the air fryer basket with non-stick baking paper and spray with olive oil. Add 4 corn dog skewers at a time and air-fry for 7–9 minutes until golden and the cheese is just melted. Turn the skewers halfway through cooking. Repeat with the second batch of skewers.

11. Let the cheese cool a little to firm up before eating as it will be really hot. Serve drizzled with your combo of favourite sauces.

KCALS per serving 138   FAT 6.6g   SAT FAT 3.5g   CARBS 12.2g   SUGARS 0.6g   FIBRE 0.4g   PROTEIN 7.2g   SALT 0.47g

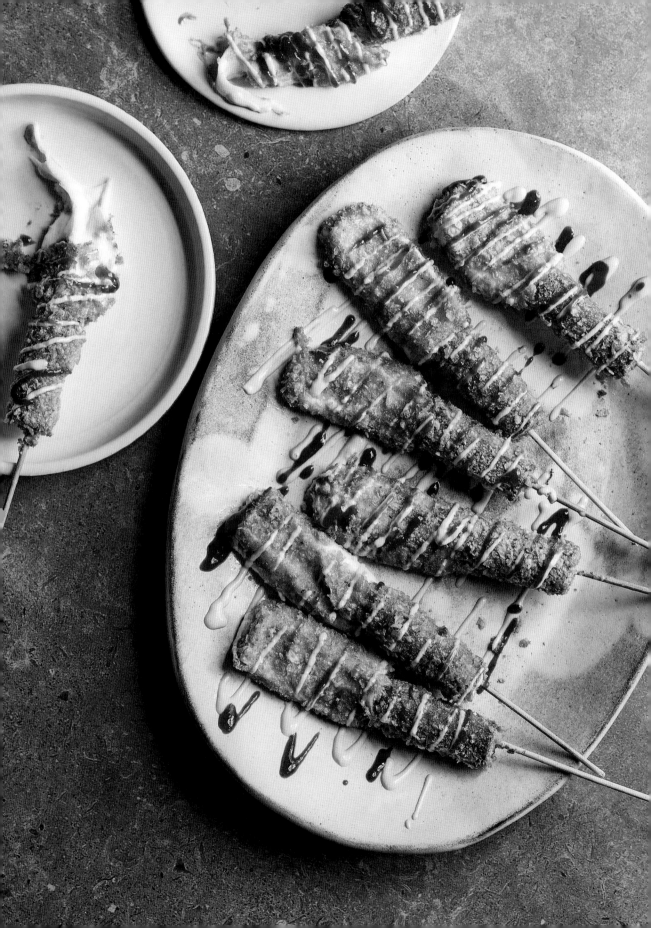

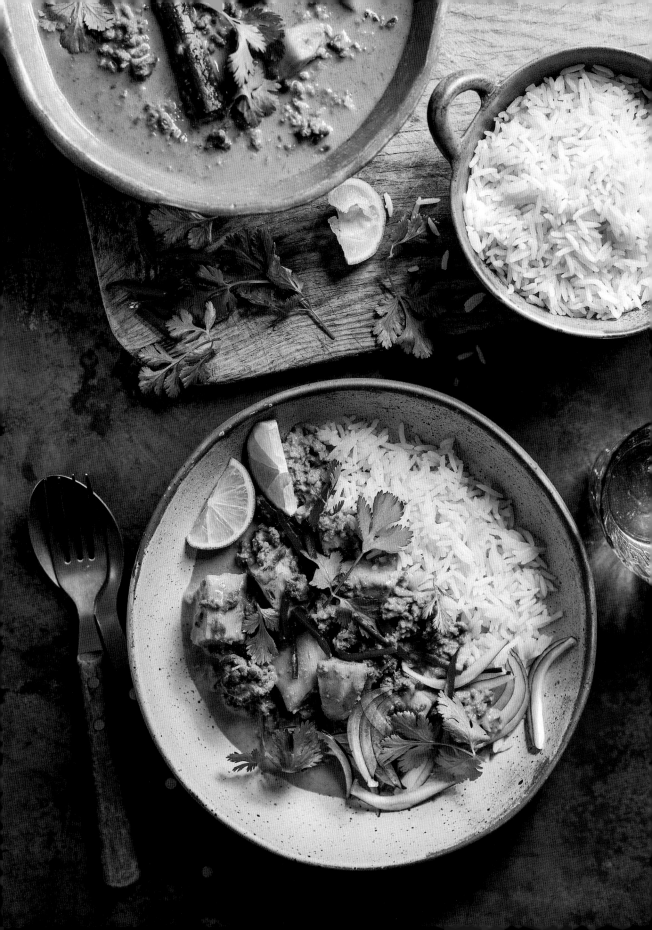

SERVES 4
PREP: **10 MINS**
COOK: **16 MINS**

RENDANG-STYLE BEEF CURRY WITH POTATOES

200g (7oz) waxy potatoes, peeled and diced

120ml (4fl oz) hot beef stock

olive oil spray

400g (14oz) 5% beef mince (ground beef)

1 tbsp cornflour (cornstarch)

1 tbsp maple syrup

4 green cardamom pods

3 whole cloves

1 whole cinnamon stick

400ml (14fl oz) light coconut milk

1 tbsp fish sauce

1 tbsp tamarind paste

salt and freshly ground black pepper

½ tsp lime zest

For the curry paste

1 onion, finely diced

1 tbsp lemongrass paste

1 tbsp grated fresh ginger

4 garlic cloves, crushed

5–8 dried red chillies to taste, soaked in hot water to soften

½ tsp ground turmeric

1 tbsp ground coriander

1 tsp ground cumin

To serve

1–2 sliced red chillies

½ small red onion, thinly sliced

handful of finely chopped fresh coriander (cilantro)

lime wedges

1. To make the paste, blitz all the ingredients in a mini food processor until well combined. If necessary, add a drop of water while pulsing, to help the ingredients blend to a paste.

2. Preheat the air fryer to 190°C/375°F for 2 minutes.

3. Place a 20cm (8in.) cake barrel in the air fryer basket and add the potatoes. Air-fry for 15 minutes, adding the stock halfway through. Cook until tender, then remove the potatoes and set aside.

4. Place the beef, cornflour, maple syrup and curry paste in the cake barrel and mix to combine. Air-fry for 5 minutes until the beef is caramelized, stirring a few times during cooking.

5. Add in the cardamom pods, cloves and cinnamon bark, along with the coconut milk, fish sauce and tamarind paste with a pinch of salt and pepper and air-fry for 10 minutes, stirring halfway through. Add the potatoes back in and air-fry for a further 2 minutes.

6. Stir in the lime zest, taste and season with more salt as needed. Top with sliced red chilli, red onion and chopped coriander and serve with lime wedges for squeezing over.

Side suggestion

A traditional rice accompaniment is perfect here.

KCALS per serving 336   FAT 13.7g   SAT FAT 8.7g   CARBS 24.9g   SUGARS 9g   FIBRE 4.4g   PROTEIN 26.2g   SALT 1.35g

500g (1lb 2oz) 5% beef
  mince (ground beef)
3 spring onions (scallions),
  finely chopped
½ tsp bicarbonate of
  soda (baking soda)
½ tsp garlic granules
1 tsp grated fresh ginger
pinch of red chilli flakes
1 tbsp soy sauce
pinch of salt and ground
  black pepper
olive oil spray

For the sauce
3 tbsp low-sodium soy sauce
3 tbsp brown sugar
2 tbsp Shaoxing wine
2 tbsp oyster sauce
4 garlic cloves, crushed
1 tsp grated fresh ginger
pinch of white pepper
½ tbsp cornflour (cornstarch)

MONGOLIAN BEEF MEATBALLS

1. Place the mince in a bowl with 1 chopped spring onion and all the remaining ingredients apart from the olive oil spray. Mix together with 2 tablespoons warm water until well combined. Spray your hands with olive oil spray and shape the mixture into approximately 20 meatballs.

2. Preheat the air fryer to 190°C/375°F for 2 minutes.

3. Line the air fryer basket with non-stick baking paper and spray with olive oil. Add the meatballs and air fry for 8–10 minutes until golden. Turn the beef halfway through cooking and respray with olive oil spray.

4. To make the sauce, whisk the ingredients except for the cornflour in a jug until well combined.

5. Remove the meatballs and the baking paper. Place a 20cm (8in.) cake barrel in the air fryer basket and add the meatballs and juices.

6. Pour the sauce over the meatballs and air-fry for a further 5 minutes.

7. Mix the cornflour with 1 tablespoon warm water, stir this into the meatballs and air-fry for a further 3–5 minutes until the sauce thickens slightly. Stir the sauce halfway through cooking to ensure the cornflour gets incorporated. If the sauce thickens too much, you can stir in a little more water to loosen.

8. Sprinkle with the remaining chopped spring onion and serve.

Optional add-ons
If you like your Mongolian beef spicy, add an extra pinch of red chilli flakes.

Side suggestions
This is perfect with rice and some additional vegetables.

Swaps
If you can't find Shaoxing wine, use dry sherry instead. You can also use chicken or turkey mince in place of the beef.

KCALS per serving 259   FAT 6.1g   SAT FAT 2.7g   CARBS 21.2g   SUGARS 16.4g   FIBRE 0.6g   PROTEIN 29.5g   SALT 2.96g

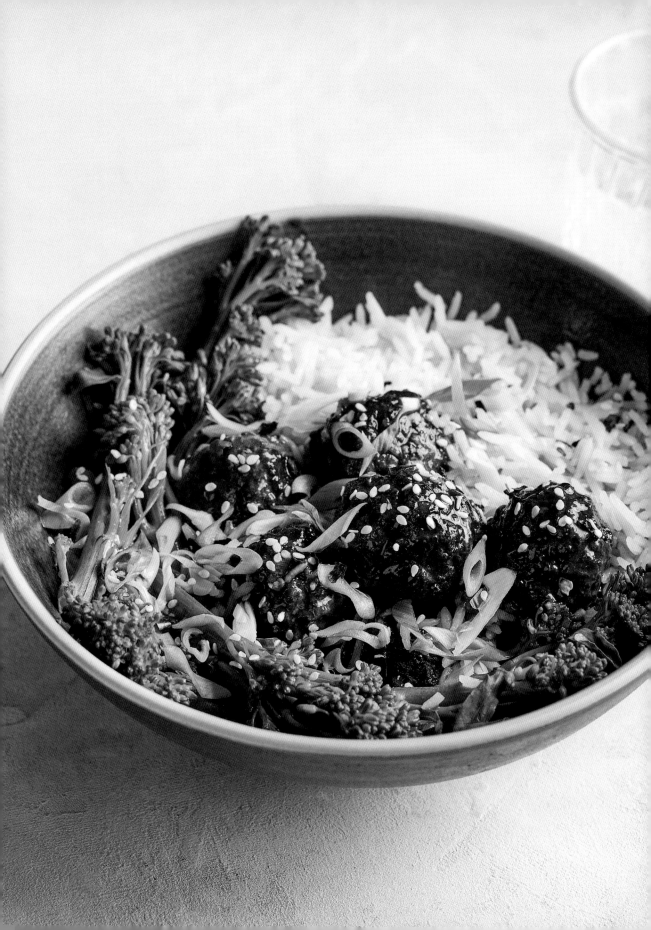

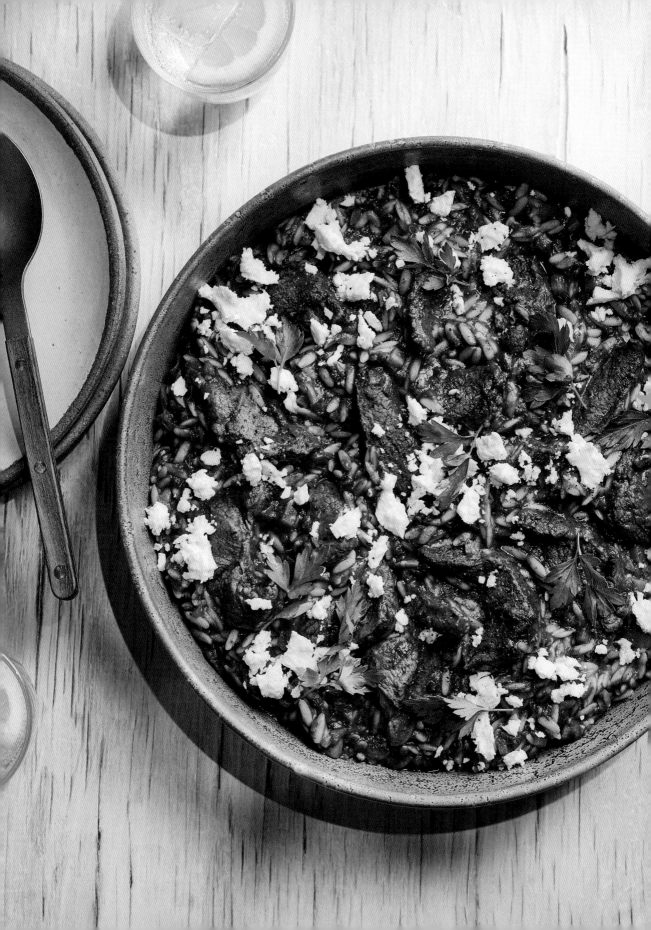

1 onion (100g/3½oz),
  finely diced

1 small carrot (80g/2¾oz),
  finely diced

olive oil spray

400g (14oz) lean lamb
  steak, sliced into strips

3 garlic cloves, crushed

1 tsp dried oregano

2 tsp sweet paprika

1 tsp dried thyme

1 tsp ground cumin

½ tsp ground cinnamon

salt and freshly ground
  black pepper

180g (6½oz) dried orzo pasta

400g (14oz) can
  chopped tomatoes in
  rich tomato juice

2 tbsp tomato purée (paste)

1 tbsp red wine vinegar

1 tsp sugar or granulated
  sweetener

480ml (16fl oz) lamb stock

50g (1¾oz) feta,
  crumbled, to serve

2 tbsp finely chopped
  fresh parsley, to serve

GREEK LAMB WITH ORZO

1. Preheat the air fryer to 200°C/400°F for 2 minutes.

2. Insert a foil/silicone liner or a 20cm (8in.) cake barrel into the air fryer basket.

3. Add in the onion and carrot and spray with olive oil spray. Air-fry for 5 minutes (if the vegetables are browning too much halfway through cooking, just add a couple of tablespoons of water).

4. Add the lamb, garlic and dried herbs and spices, along with a pinch of salt and black pepper, and stir until the lamb is completely coated in the seasonings. Air-fry for 5–6 minutes, until lightly golden around the edges.

5. Stir in the orzo, then add the tomatoes, tomato purée, red wine vinegar, sugar and stock and stir until well combined. Reduce the air fryer temperature to 190°C/375°F and air-fry for 25 minutes, stirring a few times to prevent it from browning too much on top (you can cover tightly with foil if necessary).

6. Serve topped with crumbled feta and parsley.

Swaps

This is traditionally served with kefalotyri cheese, but I use feta as a substitute. You can also use Parmesan as an alternative. Chicken stock is an option instead of lamb stock, if you prefer.

KCALS per serving 414   FAT 12.3g   SAT FAT 5.4g   CARBS 34.8g   SUGARS 9.2g   FIBRE 5.1g   PROTEIN 38.4g   SALT 0.54g

BEEF, CHORIZO AND SUN-DRIED TOMATO RAGÙ WITH PAPPARDELLE

1 onion, finely diced

1 small celery stalk, finely diced

1 small carrot, peeled and finely diced

50g (1¾oz) chorizo, diced

olive oil spray

60g (2oz) sun-dried tomatoes in oil, drained and chopped

455g (1lb) extra lean beef mince (ground beef)

3 garlic cloves, crushed

salt and freshly ground black pepper

400g (14oz) can plum tomatoes

240g (8½oz) passata

4 tbsp tomato purée (paste)

240ml (8½fl oz) hot beef stock

1 tsp Italian herb seasoning

2–3 tsp granulated sweetener

1 small piece of Parmesan rind (it adds an amazing flavour to the sauce)

250g (9oz) dried pappardelle pasta

1. Preheat the air fryer to 190°C/375°F for 3 minutes.

2. Place the onion, celery, carrot and chorizo directly into the air fryer basket and spray with olive oil spray. Air-fry for 8 minutes, stirring halfway to ensure the vegetables and chorizo don't burn.

3. Add the sun-dried tomatoes, beef mince and garlic with a good pinch of salt and black pepper. Air-fry for 10 minutes, stirring halfway through cooking to break up any large lumps and ensure that the meat is evenly cooked.

4. Transfer everything to a 20cm (8in.) cake barrel. Add the plum tomatoes, passata, tomato purée (paste), stock, Italian herb seasoning and sweetener and stir into the beef to combine.

5. Drop in the Parmesan rind and cover tightly with foil. Air-fry for 25 minutes on 190°C/375°F. Stir the beef and remove the foil for the final 10 minutes of cooking.

6. Cook the pappardelle according to the packet instructions until al dente.

7. Remove the Parmesan rind from the meat sauce and serve the ragù over the pappardelle.

<u>Optional add-ons</u>

Grate some additional fresh Parmesan over the top when serving.

KCALS per serving 566   FAT 11.5g   SAT FAT 4.4g   CARBS 68g   SUGARS 18.9g   FIBRE 9.4g   PROTEIN 42.7g   SALT 0.95g

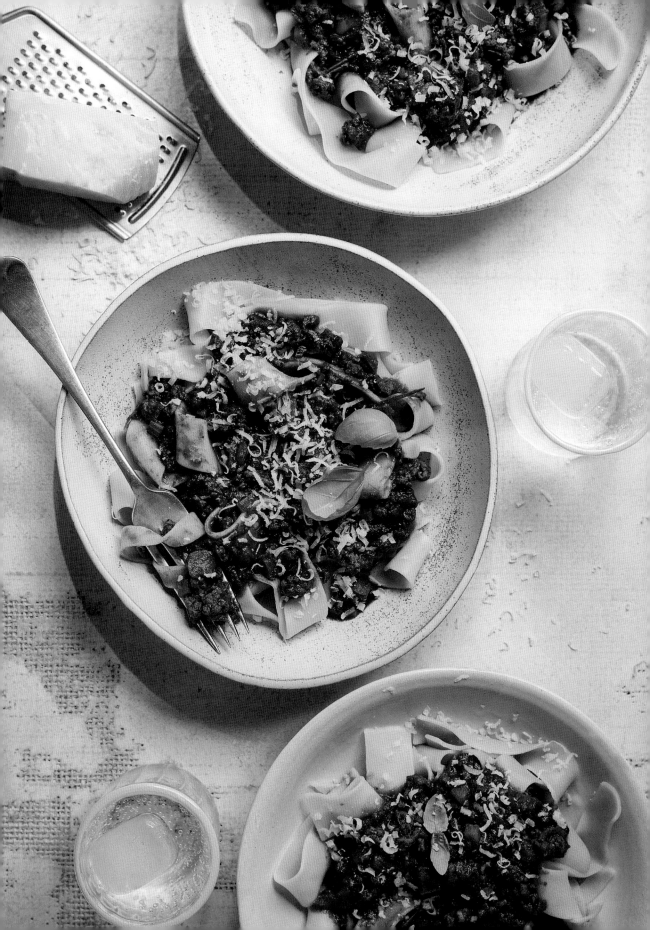

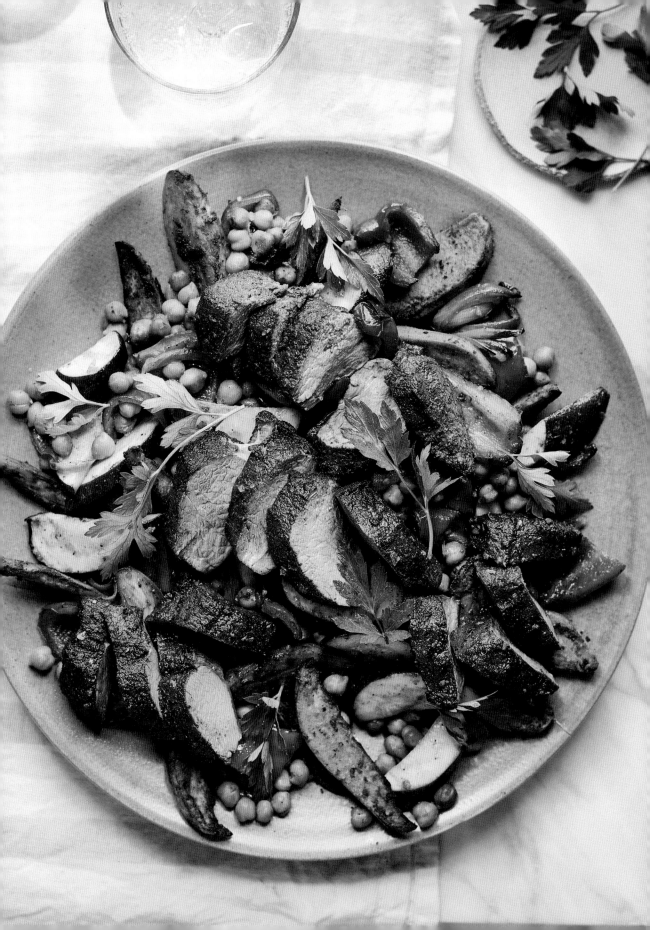

RAS EL HANOUT LAMB CHOPS WITH SWEET POTATO AND CHICKPEAS

4 lamb loin chops, trimmed of visible fat or lamb fillet (approx. 350g/12oz)

1½ tbsp ras el hanout seasoning

300g (10½oz) sweet potatoes, peeled and sliced into wedges (not too large)

½ tbsp extra virgin olive oil

1 tsp garlic granules

1½ tsp sweet paprika

salt and freshly ground black pepper

olive oil spray

200g (7oz) canned chickpeas, drained

½ tsp onion granules

½ tbsp maple syrup

130g (4½ oz) courgettes (zucchii), halved and sliced

½ green (bell) pepper, chopped

½ red (bell) pepper, chopped

½ red onion, sliced

100ml (3½fl oz) hot chicken stock

handful of finely chopped fresh coriander (cilantro), to serve

1. Remove the lamb from the fridge approximately 30 minutes before cooking to allow the chops to come to room temperature.

2. Rub the ras el hanout over the lamb until it is completely coated. Set aside to marinate.

3. Place the sweet potato wedges in a bowl with the olive oil, ½ teaspoon garlic granules, ½ teaspoon paprika and a good pinch of salt and pepper and toss to coat.

4. Place the sweet potatoes directly in the air fryer basket (or use a foil/silicone liner that fits). Air-fry at 190°C/375°F for 15 minutes. Turn the potatoes halfway through cooking and spray with olive oil spray. Remove and set aside.

5. While the sweet potatoes are cooking, place the drained chickpeas in a bowl and combine with the remaining paprika, garlic granules, onion granules and maple syrup and toss to coat.

6. Preheat the air fryer to 200°C/400°F for 2 minutes.

7. Place the lamb chops (or fillet) in the air fryer and scatter the courgettes, peppers and red onion in between, spray over the top with olive oil spray and air-fry for 9–10 minutes.

8. Halfway through cooking, turn the lamb and scatter over the chickpeas. Pour in the stock and spray over the top with some more olive oil spray.

9. Remove the lamb and rest for 5 minutes. Push the chickpeas and vegetables to one side of the basket, add the sweet potato back in and reduce the heat to 190°C/375°F. Air-fry for 3 minutes.

10. Slice the lamb and serve with the sweet potato, chickpeas and veg and a scattering of fresh coriander.

<u>Topping suggestion</u>

Delicious served with a dollop of Greek yoghurt.

KCALS per serving 594 FAT 19.5g SAT FAT 6.8g CARBS 52.4g SUGARS 17.6g FIBRE 14.5g PROTEIN 44.9g SALT 1.04g

PEANUT BUTTER AND JALAPEÑO RASPBERRY JAM BURGERS

4 tbsp reduced sugar raspberry jam (jelly), preferably seedless

30g (1oz) pickled jalapeños, finely chopped

400g (14oz) 5% beef mince (ground beef)

2 slices of lean bacon (approx 50g/1¾oz), fat removed, finely chopped

½ tsp garlic granules

½ tsp onion granules

salt and freshly ground black pepper

olive oil spray

1 red onion, halved and sliced

4 low-calorie wholemeal buns (60g/2oz each)

80g (2½oz) shredded lettuce

4 light cheese slices

4 tbsp crunchy peanut butter (natural)

gherkin (pickle) slices, to serve (optional)

1. Mix the jam and pickled jalapeños together in a bowl and set aside.

2. Place the beef in a separate bowl and add the bacon and garlic and onion granules with a pinch of salt and pepper. Mix thoroughly to combine. Spray your hands with olive oil spray and shape the mixture into 4 burgers.

3. Preheat the air fryer to 190°C/375°F for 2 minutes.

4. Line the air fryer basket with non-stick baking paper or use the grill pan insert. Spray with olive oil spray.

5. Add the burgers, scatter the onion in between and spray over the top with olive oil spray. Air-fry for 12 minutes, turning the burgers halfway through cooking and spraying with more olive oil spray.

6. Split the burger buns and lightly toast them in a pan over a medium heat, then remove and start assembling the burgers. Add lettuce to the bottom half of the bun and add the burger with a cheese slice. Spoon over the peanut butter, jalapeño jam, caramelized onion and sliced gherkin (if you like), and top with the other half of the bun.

KCALS per serving 479   FAT 17.5g   SAT FAT 5.5g   CARBS 37.5g   SUGARS 10.9g   FIBRE 6.2g   PROTEIN 39.6g   SALT 2.01g

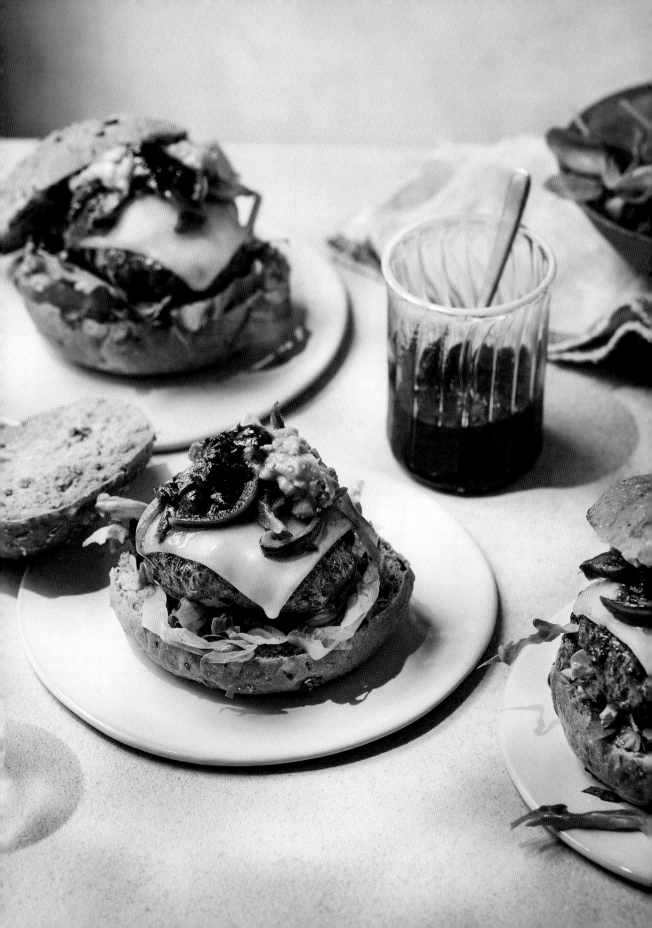

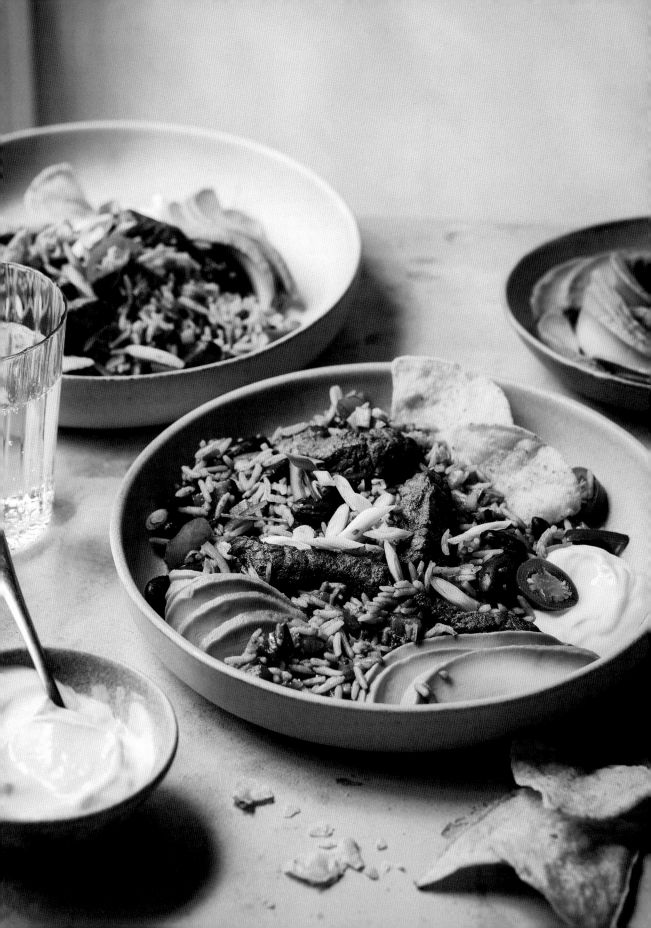

CHILLI COFFEE STEAK WITH RICE

180g (6½oz) long-grain rice, uncooked

350g (12oz) sirloin (or your steak of choice), trimmed of visible fat and sliced into strips

1 tbsp sweet paprika

2 tsp ground cumin

1 tsp dried oregano

1 tsp garlic granules

1 tsp onion granules

½ tsp cayenne pepper

1 tbsp soy sauce

olive oil spray

½ red (bell) pepper, diced

½ green (bell) pepper, diced

1 onion, diced

120ml (4fl oz) brewed black coffee

1 tbsp brown granulated sweetener

3 garlic cloves, crushed

260ml (8½fl oz) hot chicken stock

400g (14oz) can kidney beans, drained

4 tbsp tomato purée (paste)

3 spring onions (scallions), chopped

1. Cook the rice in advance (preferably the day before) and chill once cooked.

2. Place the beef in a bowl. Add the herbs and spices along with the soy sauce and mix well to combine.

3. Preheat the air fryer to 200°C/400°F for 3 minutes.

4. Place the steak directly into the air fryer basket or use a foil/silicone liner that fits. Spray with olive oil spray. Add the (bell) peppers and onion and cook for 5 minutes.

5. Stir in the coffee, brown granulated sweetener and garlic until well combined and air-fry for a further 5 minutes.

6. Add in the stock, kidney beans, tomato purée, spring onion and chilled cooked rice and stir until everything is well combined. Air-fry for a final 5–8 minutes until most of the liquid is absorbed and just loosely coats everything.

7. Serve with your favourite toppings (see Topping suggestions below).

Topping suggestions

Guacamole or avocado, soured cream, Cheddar, sliced jalapeños, coriander (cilantro), diced tomatoes, chopped spring onions. This dish is also great with a few nacho chips.

KCALS per serving 430 FAT 5.8g SAT FAT 2.1g CARBS 57g SUGARS 7.4g FIBRE 9.7g PROTEIN 32.5g SALT 1.11g

BEEF NOODLE STIR-FRY

400g (14oz) steak of your choice, trimmed of visible fat and thinly sliced

½ tsp bicarbonate of soda (baking soda)

1 tsp dark soy sauce

olive oil spray

1 red (bell) pepper, sliced

1 onion, sliced

200g (7oz) dried egg noodles

300g (10½oz) pak choi, roughly chopped

3 spring onions (scallions), chopped

pinch of freshly ground black pepper

For the sauce

2 tbsp light soy sauce

2 tbsp dark soy sauce

2 garlic cloves, crushed

thumb-sized piece of fresh ginger, thinly sliced

2 tbsp apricot jam

1 tbsp honey

1 tsp sesame oil

1 tbsp rice vinegar

2 tsp sriracha

1. Place the beef in a bowl and sprinkle with the bicarbonate of soda. Toss to coat and leave to sit for approximately 15 minutes (but no longer). Add the dark soy sauce and toss again.

2. To make the sauce, place the dark and light soy sauces in a separate bowl. Add the garlic, ginger, apricot jam, honey, sesame oil, rice vinegar and sriracha and whisk to combine, then set aside.

3. Preheat the air fryer to 200°C/400°F for 3 minutes.

4. Place the beef directly into the air fryer basket. Spray over the top with olive oil spray and air-fry for 2–3 minutes until browned. Once cooked, remove and set aside, leaving some of the juices in the pan.

5. Add the (bell) pepper and onion, spray with olive oil spray and air-fry for 5 minutes until tender.

6. While the vegetables are cooking, place the egg noodles in a large bowl and cover with boiling water. Place a plate over the bowl and leave for 5 minutes, then drain and spray with some olive oil spray. Toss to coat and set aside.

7. Add the pak choi and spring onion to the (bell) peppers and onion, spray with olive oil spray and stir to coat. Air-fry for 1 minute.

8. Add the beef and sauce back in, turn to coat and air-fry for 2 minutes.

9. Add the noodles, mix until everything is well combined and cook for a final 2 minutes, then season with a pinch of black pepper and serve.

Tip

You can increase the sriracha if you prefer a spicier dish.

KCALS per serving 428 FAT 7.3g SAT FAT 2.4g CARBS 55g SUGARS 19.1g FIBRE 5.4g PROTEIN 32.8g SALT 3.7g

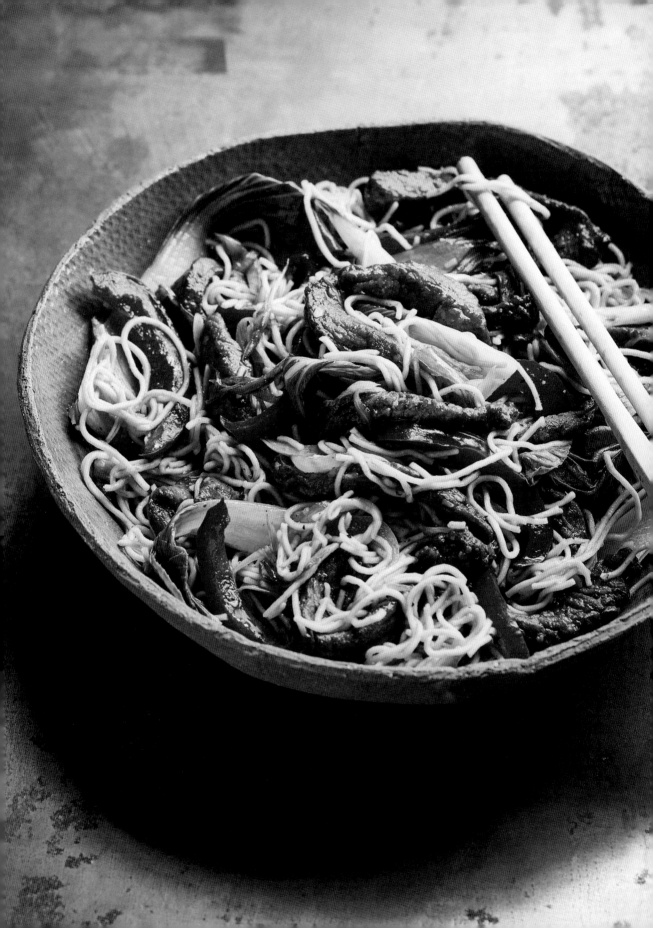

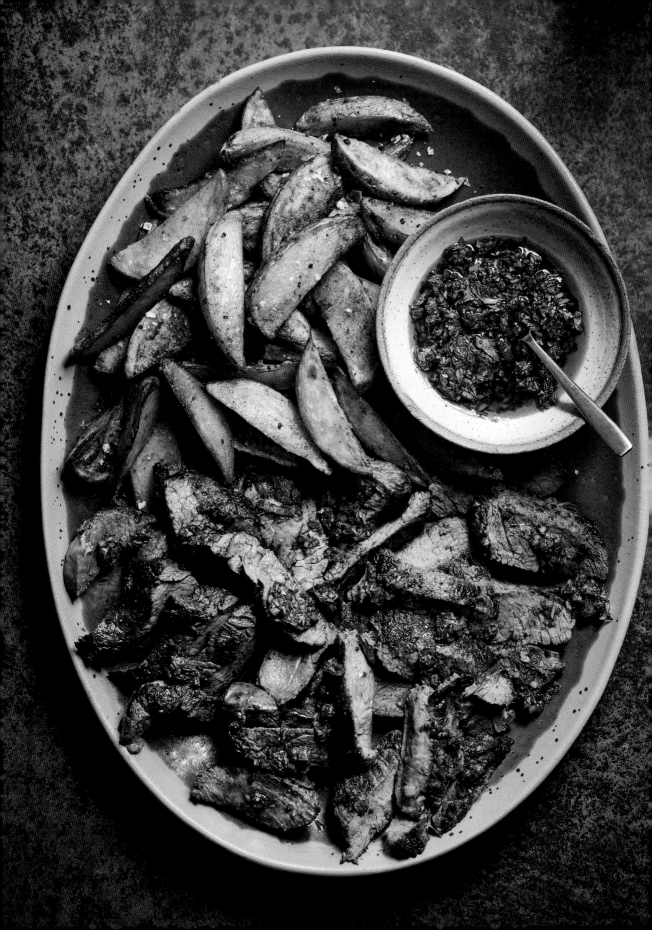

SERVES 4
PREP: **15 MINS**
COOK: **30 MINS**

SEASONED STEAK WITH CHIMICHURRI SAUCE AND GARLIC WEDGES

4 steaks of your choice, trimmed of visible fat (160g/5¾oz) per person)
pinch of ground black pepper
½ tsp garlic granules
½ tsp onion granules
¾ tsp coarse sea salt
olive oil spray

For the garlic potato wedges
800g (28oz) floury potatoes, skin on, sliced into thin wedges
1 tsp garlic granules
½ tsp onion granules
½ tsp sweet paprika
¾ tsp salt
pinch of ground black pepper
olive oil spray

For the chimichurri sauce
4 tbsp finely chopped fresh parsley
2 tbsp finely chopped fresh coriander (cilantro)
2 garlic cloves, crushed
1 shallot, finely diced
½ tsp Italian herb seasoning
½ tsp sweet paprika
¼ tsp coarse sea salt
pinch of black pepper
1 small red chilli (seeds removed), diced
1 tbsp extra virgin olive oil
1 tbsp red wine vinegar
1 tbsp fresh lime juice

1. To prepare the garlic potatoes, place the potato wedges in a bowl and cover with water. Drop in some ice cubes and leave to soak for at least 30 minutes.

2. To make the chimichurri sauce, mix all the ingredients together in a small bowl with 1 tablespoon water. Set aside to allow the flavours to develop.

3. Remove the steaks from the fridge at least 20 minutes before cooking. Rub them all over with the black pepper and garlic and onion granules and season both sides generously with coarse sea salt.

4. Drain the potatoes, pat them dry with a clean paper towel and place them in a bowl. Add the garlic and onion granules, paprika, salt and a good pinch of black pepper. Spray with olive oil spray, toss and then spray again to coat.

5. Preheat the air fryer to 200°C/400°F for 2 minutes.

6. Line the air fryer basket with non-stick baking paper or use the grill pan insert. Spray with olive oil spray. Add the potato wedges and air-fry for 20 minutes until golden. Turn the potatoes halfway through cooking and spray again with olive oil spray. Remove and set aside.

7. Preheat the air fryer to 200°C/400°F for 3–5 minutes (it needs to be really hot before you add the steaks).

8. Place the steaks in the air fryer, spray with olive oil spray and cook for 8–10 minutes, depending on thickness. This should result in medium-rare – cook for longer if you prefer it cooked to medium/well done (though chimichurri steak is best served medium-rare).

9. Rest the steaks for 8–10 minutes, then slice them thinly against the grain. While the steaks are resting you can add the potatoes back in to reheat, then adjust the seasoning to taste.

10. Serve the steak slices, drizzled with the chimichurri sauce, with the potato wedges and additional greens (if you like).

KCALS per serving 439   FAT 11.3g   SAT FAT 3.9g   CARBS 39.3g   SUGARS 2.4g   FIBRE 5.1g   PROTEIN 42.7g   SALT 2.35g

FIRE MEATBALLS WITH CHEESE

500g (1lb 2oz) 5% fat beef mince (ground beef)
½ tsp bicarbonate of soda (baking soda)
1 spring onion (scallion), chopped
1 tbsp soy sauce
½ tsp onion granules
½ tsp garlic granules
pinch of salt and ground black pepper
olive oil spray
100g (3½oz) mozzarella, torn into pieces
2 spring onions (scallions), chopped, to serve

For the sauce
2 tbsp gochujang
2 tbsp maple syrup
1 tbsp tomato purée (paste)
1 tbsp soy sauce
2 garlic cloves, crushed
½ tbsp finely grated fresh ginger
1 tsp sesame oil

1. To make the sauce, whisk all the ingredients along with 120ml (4fl oz) water in a jug. Set aside.

2. Place the beef in a bowl with the bicarbonate of soda, spring onion, soy sauce, onion and garlic granules, salt and pepper and mix with 2 tablespoons water until all the ingredients are combined. Spray your hands with the olive oil spray and shape the mixture into approximately 16 meatballs.

3. Preheat the air fryer to 190°C/375°F.

4. Line the air fryer basket with non-stick baking paper and spray with olive oil spray. Add the meatballs and air-fry for 8 minutes. Turn the meatballs halfway through cooking and spray again with olive oil spray.

5. Transfer the meatballs (and any juices) to a 20cm (8in.) cake barrel and pour over the sauce. Remove the non-stick baking paper from the air fryer basket and place the cake barrel in the air fryer. Air-fry for 5 minutes.

6. Scatter the mozzarella over the top, reduce the temperature to 180°C/350°F and air-fry for a further 3–4 minutes until the cheese is melted and lightly golden on top.

7. Sprinkle with the chopped spring onions and serve.

Serving suggestions
Serve with rice and sliced cucumber (the cucumber helps to balance the heat).

Dairy-free
These are equally delicious without the cheese.

KCALS per serving 292   FAT 12.9g   SAT FAT 6.4g   CARBS 12.6g   SUGARS 8.7g   FIBRE 0.8g   PROTEIN 31g   SALT 2.19g

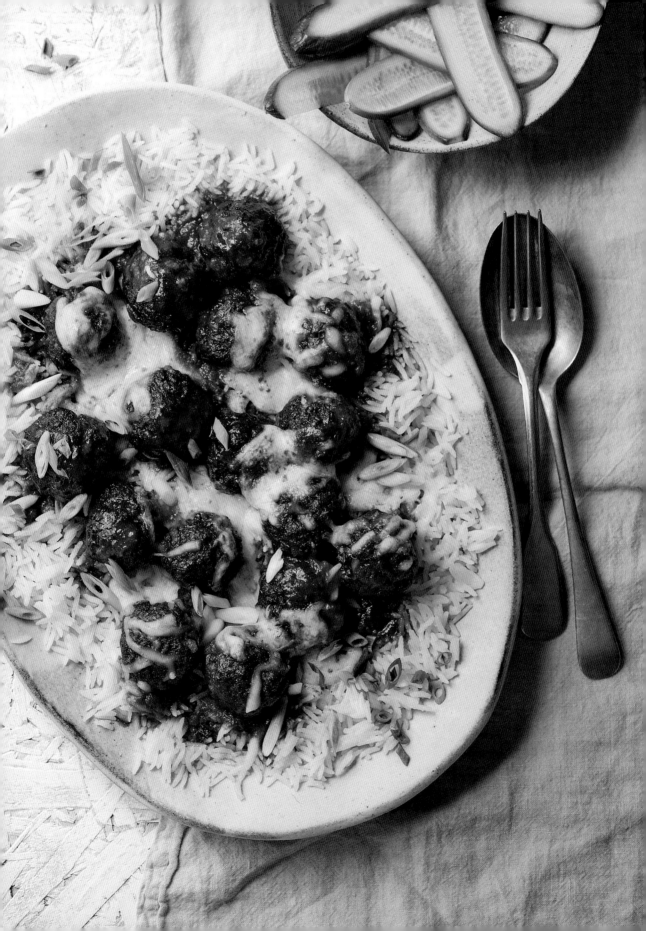

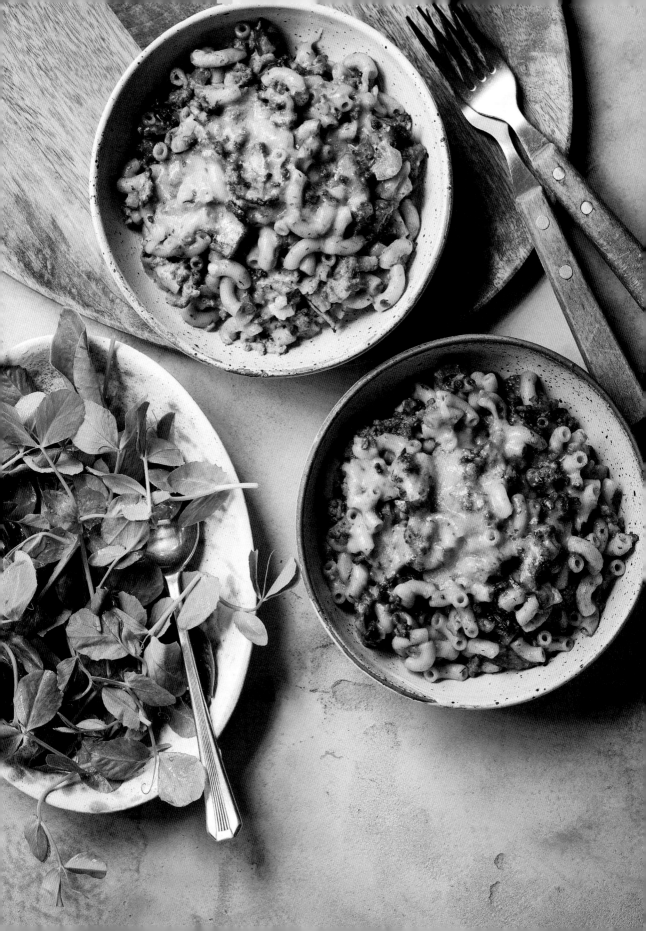

CHIPOTLE BEEF MACARONI

250g (9oz) dried
  macaroni pasta

olive oil spray

1 onion, finely diced

½ red (bell) pepper, diced

½ green (bell) pepper, diced

70g lean bacon, trimmed
  of visible fat, chopped

455g (1lb) 5% fat beef
  mince (ground beef)

2 garlic cloves, crushed
  (70g/2½oz)

1 tsp sweet paprika

1 tsp garlic granules

1 tsp onion granules

1 tsp dried dill

1 tsp dried parsley

½ tsp smoked paprika

2 tbsp light cream cheese

180ml (6fl oz) hot
  chicken stock

1 tbsp tomato purée (paste)

2 tbsp chipotle paste

180ml (6fl oz) semi-
  skimmed milk

1 tbsp cornflour (cornstarch)

100g (3½oz) Cheddar, grated

1. Cook the pasta according to the packet instructions until al dente. Reserve 80ml (3fl oz) of the pasta cooking water and set aside. Drain the pasta and spray with olive oil spray (this will prevent the pasta from sticking together). Toss to coat and set aside.

2. While the pasta is cooking, preheat the air fryer to 200°C/400°F for 2 minutes.

3. Place the onion and (bell) peppers directly into the air fryer basket or use a foil/silicone liner that fits and spray with olive oil spray. Air-fry for 5 minutes until the vegetables are slightly softened.

4. Reduce the heat to 190°C/375°F, stir in the bacon, beef mince and garlic and air-fry for 4 minutes. Add in the seasonings and mix until all coated, then continue to cook for an additional 3–4 minutes until the mince is cooked.

5. In a jug, stir the cream cheese into the hot stock until melted, then add to the beef along with the tomato purée and chipotle paste.

6. Combine the milk with the cornflour and add this too. Air-fry for another 5 minutes.

7. Stir in the cooked pasta, reserved pasta water and Cheddar until well combined and air-fry for a couple more minutes until the sauce around the beef and pasta is all creamy and cheesy.

Side suggestions

Pair with some additional side vegetables or a salad.

KCALS per serving 592   FAT 17.6g   SAT FAT 9.1g   CARBS 57.5g   SUGARS 8.8g   FIBRE 5.9g   PROTEIN 47.9g   SALT 1.9g

600g (21oz) sirloin (or your steak of choice), trimmed of visible fat and cubed

200g (7oz) button mushrooms, halved

1 small red onion, sliced

1 green (bell) pepper, sliced

olive oil spray

For the marinade

2 tbsp low-sodium soy sauce

2 garlic cloves, crushed

1 tbsp Worcestershire sauce

1 tbsp balsamic vinegar

1 tbsp maple syrup

1 tsp Dijon mustard

For the Montreal steak seasoning

1 tsp sweet paprika

1 tsp garlic granules

½ tsp onion granules

½ tsp dried dill

½ tsp ground coriander

½ tsp freshly ground black pepper

½ tsp sea salt

pinch of chilli flakes

MONTREAL STEAK BITE SKEWERS

1. To make the marinade, whisk the ingredients together in a jug until well combined.

2. Place the steak in a bag or container, cover with the marinade and refrigerate overnight.

3. Mix the steak seasoning ingredients together in a bowl until well combined.

4. Remove the steak from the marinade, discarding any excess marinade, and toss in the seasoning until well coated.

5. Thread the steak pieces, mushrooms, red onion and green (bell) pepper onto metal skewers (first make sure these fit in your air fryer).

6. Preheat the air fryer to 200°C/400°F for 5 minutes (this is vital).

7. Line the air fryer basket with non-stick baking paper or use the grill pan insert. Spray with olive oil spray. Add the skewers and air-fry for 6 minutes. Turn the skewers halfway through cooking and respray with a little olive oil spray. If you like your steak pieces well done, cook for a further 2 minutes.

Serving suggestions

These are great with a salad, potato wedges, rice, or on a pita bread/flatbread.

KCALS per serving 262   FAT 7.8g   SAT FAT 3.1g   CARBS 8.6g   SUGARS 6.4g   FIBRE 1.9g   PROTEIN 38.3g   SALT 1.86g

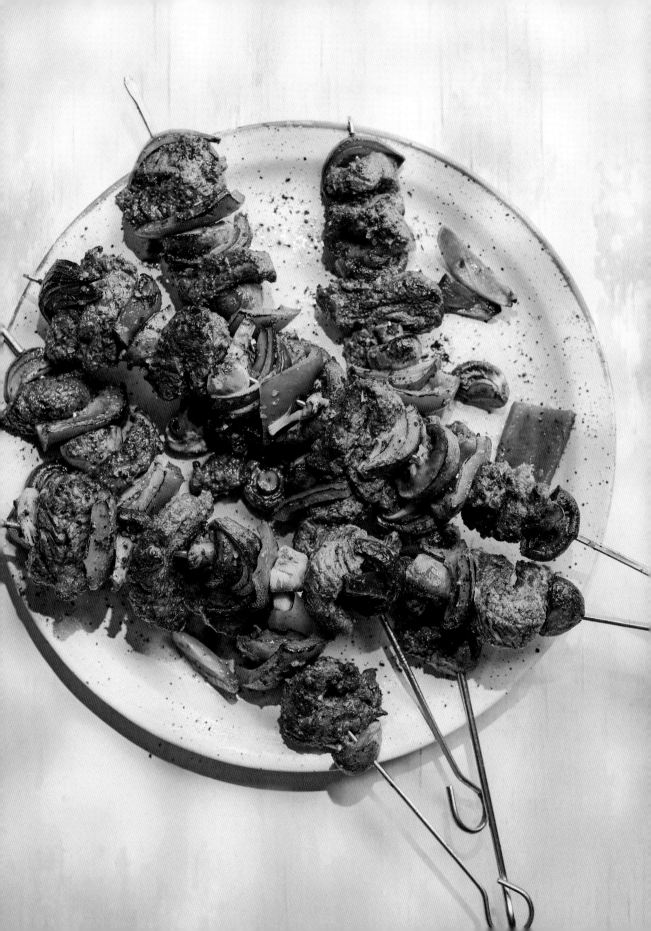

THE ULTIMATE CHEESEBURGER CHIMICHANGAS

olive oil spray

455g (1lb) 5% fat beef mince (ground beef)

½ onion, finely diced

100g (3½oz) ripe tomato, cored, seeded and finely diced

1 tsp sweet paprika

1 tsp garlic granules

pinch of salt and freshly ground black pepper

2 tsp American yellow mustard

2 tbsp tomato purée (paste)

½ tbsp Worcestershire sauce

4 low-calorie 20cm (8in.) white tortilla wraps

125g (4½oz) chopped gherkins (pickles)

120g (4¼oz) Cheddar slices

For the burger sauce

3 tbsp light mayonnaise

1 tbsp fat-free Greek yogurt

1 tsp tomato purée (paste)

1 tsp American yellow mustard

½ tsp sweet paprika

¼ tsp garlic granules

¼ tsp onion granules

pinch of ground black pepper

1 tsp granulated sweetener (optional)

1. To make the burger sauce, whisk all the ingredients in a jug and add a little water to loosen.

2. Preheat the air fryer to 200°C/400°F for 3 minutes.

3. Line the air fryer basket with non-stick baking paper or use the grill pan insert. Spray with olive oil spray. Add the mince, onion, tomato and seasonings and air-fry for 10 minutes until cooked. Stir halfway through cooking.

4. Transfer to a bowl and stir in the mustard, tomato purée and Worcestershire sauce.

5. Place a quarter of the beef in the middle of a wrap, sprinkle with the chopped gherkin, then top with the cheese. Fold in the sides and then tightly roll into a wrap. Repeat with the rest of the beef until you have 4 filled wraps.

6. Spray the air fryer basket with olive oil spray. Add the wraps, seam-side down, to the air fryer basket (or use the grill pan insert if your air fryer has one) and air-fry for approximately 4 minutes at 190°C/375°F. Turn and air-fry for another 4 minutes until golden brown all over (all the chimichangas should be cooked at the same time, not individually).

7. Serve the chimichangas on some shredded lettuce. Drizzle some burger sauce over the top and then sprinkle with some chopped onion, gherkins, tomatoes and pickled jalapeño, if you like.

Swaps

You can use American processed cheese slices if you prefer.

KCALS per serving 494   FAT 20g   SAT FAT 9.5g   CARBS 34.5g   SUGARS 7.7g   FIBRE 9.3g   PROTEIN 39.4g   SALT 1.83g

To serve

1 head of romaine or ½ small iceberg lettuce, shredded

1 small onion, diced

12 gherkin (pickle) slices, chopped

1 ripe tomato (core and seeds removed)

pickled jalapeño slices (optional)

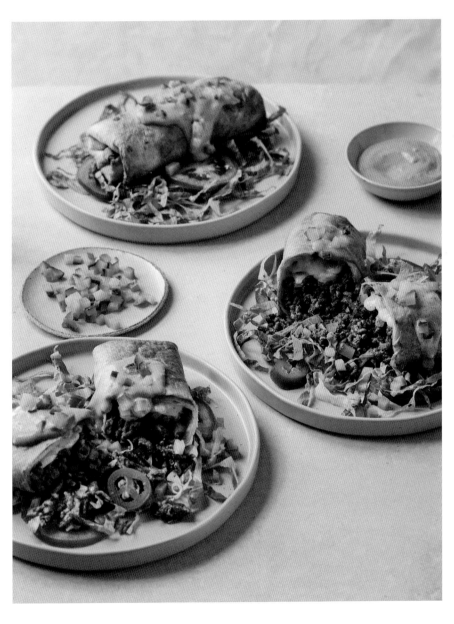

PERSIAN-STYLE LAMB HOTPOT

650g (23oz) floury
 potatoes (skin on),
 sliced into thin rounds

1 onion, finely diced

olive oil spray

455g (1lb) lean lamb
 mince (ground lamb)

2 garlic cloves, crushed

1 tbsp honey

1 tsp ground cumin

1 tsp ground turmeric

½ tsp chilli powder or
 cayenne pepper

½ tsp ground coriander

¼ tsp ground nutmeg

¼ tsp ground cinnamon

salt and freshly ground
 black pepper

4 tbsp tomato purée (paste)

160ml (5½fl oz) hot
 chicken stock

2 tsp cornflour (cornstarch)

1 tbsp finely chopped
 fresh parsley

1 tbsp finely chopped fresh
 coriander (cilantro)

handful of finely chopped
 fresh coriander

5 tbsp fat-free Greek yogurt

seeds from ½ pomegranate

1. Bring a large saucepan of water to a boil, add the potatoes and parboil for 5–6 minutes until just tender.

2. Preheat the air fryer to 190°C/375°F for 2 minutes.

3. Place the onion directly into the air fryer basket or use a foil/silicone liner that fits. Spray with olive oil spray and air-fry for 5 minutes.

4. Add in the lamb, garlic, honey, cumin, turmeric, chilli powder, coriander, nutmeg and cinnamon with half the tomato purée, season with a pinch of salt and black pepper and mix to combine. Flatten the lamb out in an even layer and cook for 5 minutes until browned.

5. Pour in 120ml (4fl oz) of the stock, cornflour, fresh parsley, fresh coriander and the remaining tomato purée and mix to combine. Transfer to a foil tray (or use an ovenproof dish that fits in the air fryer basket).

6. Drain the potatoes, spray with olive oil spray and toss to coat.

7. Lay the potatoes over the meat mixture so that they are slightly overlapping and pour the remaining stock over the top.

8. Set the air fryer temperature to 180°C/350°F and cook for 20–30 minutes until the potatoes are lightly golden and cooked through. Cover the tray tightly with foil if the potatoes begin to brown too much on top.

9. Sprinkle with fresh coriander and serve with a dollop of Greek yogurt and some pomegranate seeds.

KCALS per serving 402   FAT 11.8g   SAT FAT 4.9g   CARBS 38.9g   SUGARS 12.3g   FIBRE 5.2g   PROTEIN 32.4g   SALT 0.46g

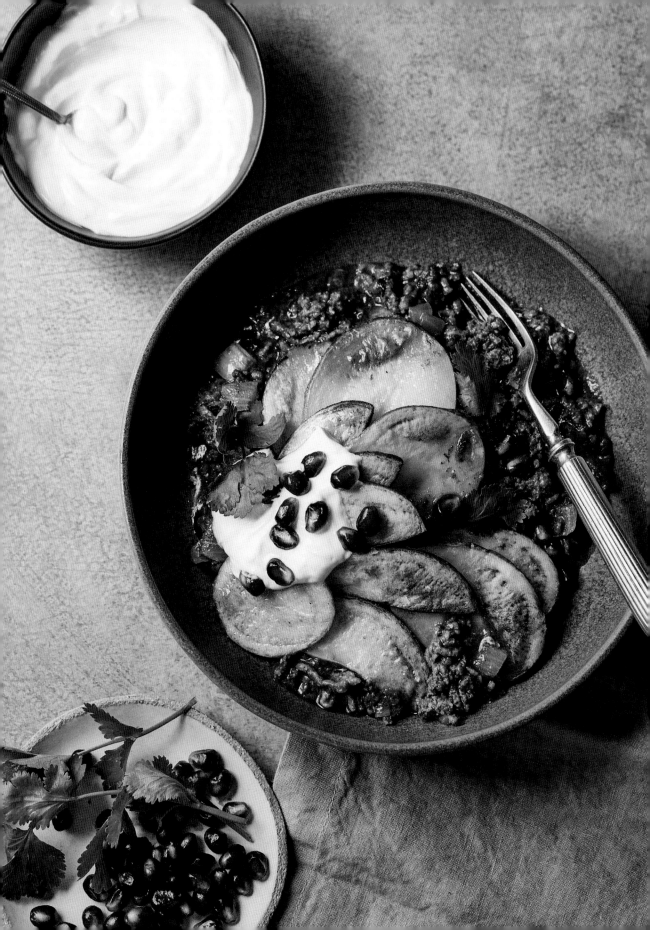

FISH AND SEAFOOD

COCONUT PANKO PRAWN
SALAD WITH LOUISIANA
REMOULADE 138

SPICY TUNA GRILLED
CHEESE BITES WITH
CUCUMBER SALAD 141

TUNA LASAGNE PIE 142

BUTTER SALMON AND
ASPARAGUS PASTA 145

CARIBBEAN PRAWN AND
PINEAPPLE SKEWERS WITH
COCONUT RICE 146

SWEET CHILLI SALMON
BITES WITH SESAME
GARLIC BROCCOLI 148

HIBACHI PRAWNS WITH
FRIED RICE 150

BOMBAY POTATO-TOPPED
PRAWN AND FISH PIE 153

FAJITA STUFFED SALMON 154

CHEESY, CREAMY COD
GRATIN WITH HERBY
CRUSHED POTATOES 157

PERUVIAN SPICED FISH
WITH CAULIFLOWER 158

COCONUT PANKO PRAWN SALAD WITH LOUISIANA REMOULADE

250g (9oz) fresh raw large
  prawns (shrimp), peeled

1 tbsp cornflour (cornstarch)

50g (1¾oz) panko
  breadcrumbs

2 tbsp unsweetened shredded
  coconut (desiccated)

1 egg, beaten

olive oil spray

salt and freshly ground
  black pepper

For the Louisiana
  remoulade

2 tbsp light mayonnaise

2 tbsp fat-free Greek yogurt

1 tbsp gherkin (pickle) vinegar

1 tsp granulated sweetener

½ tsp dried parsley

½ tsp dried chives

½ tsp sweet paprika

¼ tsp garlic granules

¼ tsp Worcestershire sauce

½ tsp hot sauce (I used
  Frank's Red Hot) or a
  pinch of cayenne pepper

To serve

1 head of romaine
  lettuce, chopped

½ red onion, thinly sliced

10 baby plum tomatoes halved

80g (2¾oz) avocado, sliced

1. To make the remoulade, whisk all the ingredients in a bowl, adding a little water to loosen. (If you want more of a kick, add in a little more hot sauce or cayenne pepper.)

2. Pat the prawns dry with paper towels and place in a bowl. Add the cornflour with a pinch of salt and black pepper and toss to coat.

3. In a shallow bowl, mix the panko with the coconut until well combined.

4. Dip a prawn into the beaten egg and then the panko/coconut mix to coat, gently pressing the breadcrumb mixture to ensure it sticks.

5. Repeat with the other prawns and transfer to a plate, then spray over the top with olive oil spray.

6. Preheat the air fryer to 180°C/350°F for 2 minutes.

7. Line the air fryer basket with non-stick baking paper and spray with olive oil spray. Add the coated prawns (not too closely together) and air-fry for 8–10 minutes until golden all over. Turn the prawns halfway through cooking and spray with more olive oil spray.

8. Serve with the romaine, red onion, tomato and avocado and drizzle with the remoulade dressing.

Note

*These can also be enjoyed as tacos in soft tortilla wraps or
hard taco shells, with the salad and drizzled with the dressing.*

KCALS per serving 487   FAT 20.7g   SAT FAT 6g   CARBS 38.6g   SUGARS 11.1g   FIBRE 12g   PROTEIN 30.7g   SALT 2.02g

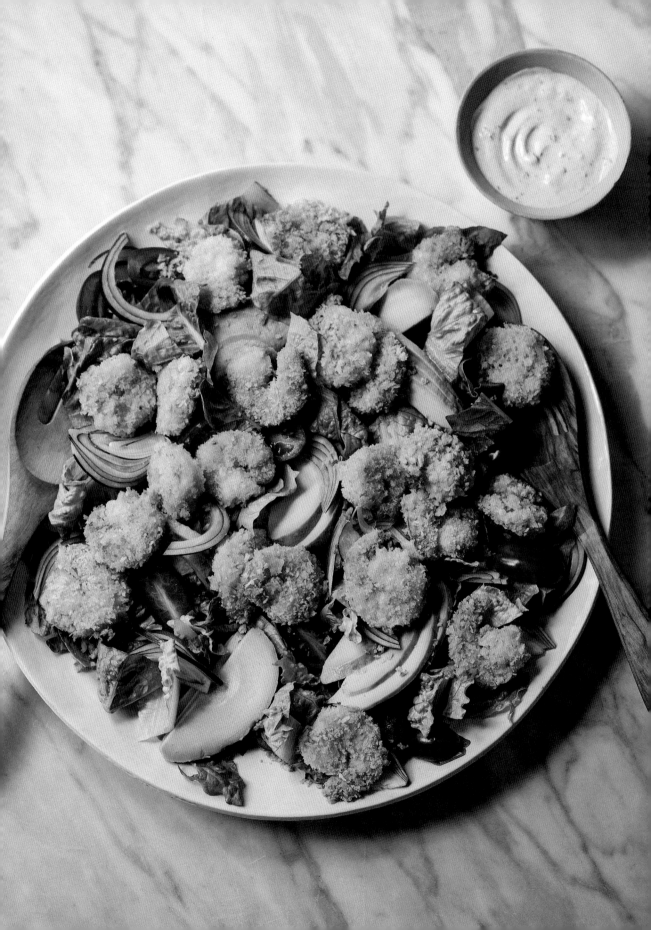

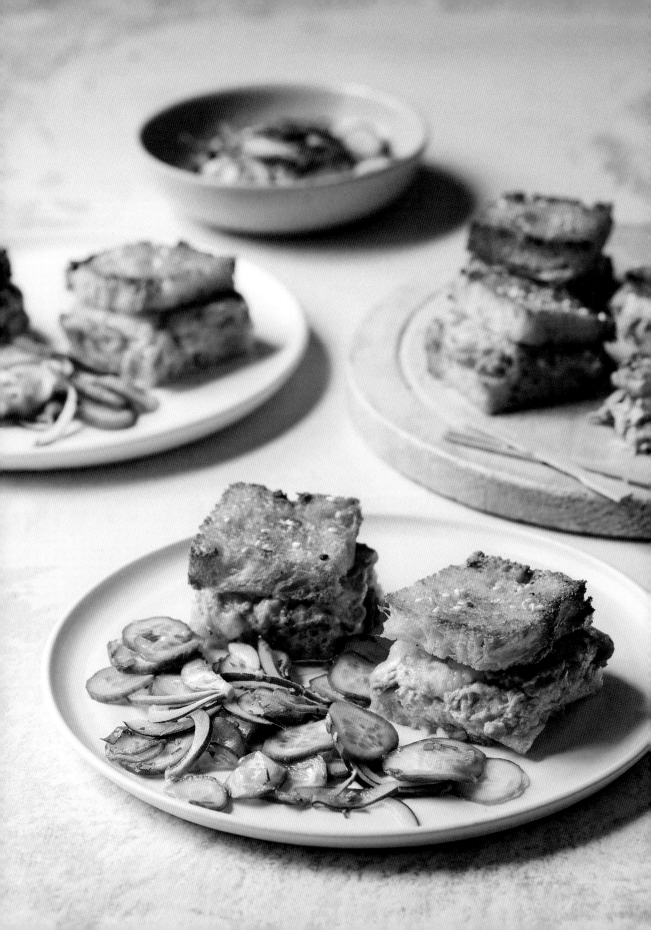

SPICY TUNA GRILLED CHEESE BITES WITH CUCUMBER SALAD

2 tbsp light mayonnaise

2 tbsp fat-free Greek yogurt

1 tbsp sriracha

145g (5oz) can tuna chunks in brine, drained

2 spring onions (scallions), sliced

salt and freshly ground black pepper

1 small avocado, mashed

¼ tsp garlic granules

1 tsp fresh lime juice

4 slices of bread, crusts removed

50g (1¾oz) mozzarella, grated

30g (1oz) Cheddar, finely grated

olive oil spray

½ tsp sesame seeds

For the salad

4 baby cucumbers, thinly sliced or ½ full-sized cucumber, thinly sliced

¼ red onion, thinly sliced

1 garlic clove, crushed

2 tbsp finely chopped fresh coriander (cilantro)

2 tbsp rice vinegar

1 tsp granulated sweetener

1. Combine all the ingredients for the cucumber salad and set aside.

2. In a bowl, mix together the mayonnaise, yogurt and sriracha, add in the tuna and spring onion and fold to combine. Season to taste with some salt and black pepper.

3. In another bowl, mash the avocado with the garlic granules and lime juice.

4. Spread the mashed avocado over two of the bread slices. Top with the tuna and then add the mozzarella and the Cheddar. Top with the other two slices of bread on top, then slice each sandwich into 4 squares, so you have 8 mini spicy tuna cheese sandwiches.

5. Preheat the air fryer to 190°C/375°F for 2 minutes.

6. Line the air fryer basket with non-stick baking paper or use the grill pan insert. Spray with olive oil spray.

7. Spray both sides of the sandwiches with olive oil spray, then place them in the basket and air-fry for approximately 4 minutes until golden on top. Turn, spray again with olive oil spray and sprinkle the top of each square with a pinch of sesame seeds. Air-fry for an additional 4 minutes (approximately) until golden.

8. Serve the cheese bites with the cucumber salad.

Tip

*Gochujang works well as a swap for the sriracha.
I make it often with either and both are yummy.*

KCALS per serving 564   FAT 28.3g   SAT FAT 9.6g   CARBS 42.2g   SUGARS 14.5g   FIBRE 5.4g   PROTEIN 32.6g   SALT 2.02g

olive oil spray
100g (3½oz) onion,
    finely diced
150g (5½oz) sweet potato,
    peeled and finely diced
½ red (bell) pepper,
    finely diced
2 garlic cloves, crushed
1 tsp sweet paprika
pinch of salt and ground
    black pepper
240g (8½oz) passata
4 tbsp tomato purée (paste)
240ml (8½fl oz) hot
    chicken stock
2 tsp granulated sweetener
85g (3oz) frozen sweetcorn,
    defrosted and drained
1 tsp Italian herb seasoning
2 x 145g (5oz) cans tuna
    in brine, drained
8 dried lasagne sheets
120g (4½oz) light
    cream cheese
3 tbsp semi-skimmed milk
pinch of garlic granules
50g (1¾oz) mozzarella, grated
60g (2oz) Cheddar, grated
salt and freshly ground
    black pepper

TUNA
LASAGNE PIE

1. Place a 20cm (8in.) cake barrel in the air fryer basket and spray with olive oil spray.

2. Preheat the air fryer to 190°C/375°F for 2 minutes.

3. Add the onion, sweet potato, (bell) pepper, garlic, paprika and a pinch of salt and black pepper to the air fryer, toss to coat and cook for 10–12 minutes until the sweet potato is tender. Stir the ingredients halfway through cooking and respray with olive oil spray.

4. Add in the passata, tomato purée, stock, sweetener, sweetcorn and Italian seasoning and air-fry for 10 minutes until the sauce thickens.

5. Fold in the tuna chunks, then transfer the tuna mix to a large bowl and clean the cake barrel.

6. Soak the lasagne sheets in boiling water for a few minutes, just to soften them so they are easier to cut.

7. Add a third of the tuna mix to the cake barrel and top with a third of the lasagne sheets, cutting them to fit the pan.

8. Add another third of the tuna mix and layer with a third of the lasagne sheets. Top with the remaining tuna mix and the last few lasagne sheets.

9. In a jug, whisk the cream cheese with the milk and garlic granules until smooth. Spread this over the top and season with salt and freshly ground black pepper.

10. Top with the mozzarella and Cheddar. Cover the cake barrel tightly with foil and air-fry for 20 minutes at 180°C/350°F, then remove the foil and air-fry for a further 10–12 minutes until the top is melted and golden. Leave to rest for 10 minutes and then slice and serve.

Side suggestion
Pair the lasagne pie with a mixed salad.

KCALS per serving 455   FAT 12.4g   SAT FAT 6.4g   CARBS 49.9g   SUGARS 12.1g   FIBRE 6.7g   PROTEIN 32.4g   SALT 1.4g

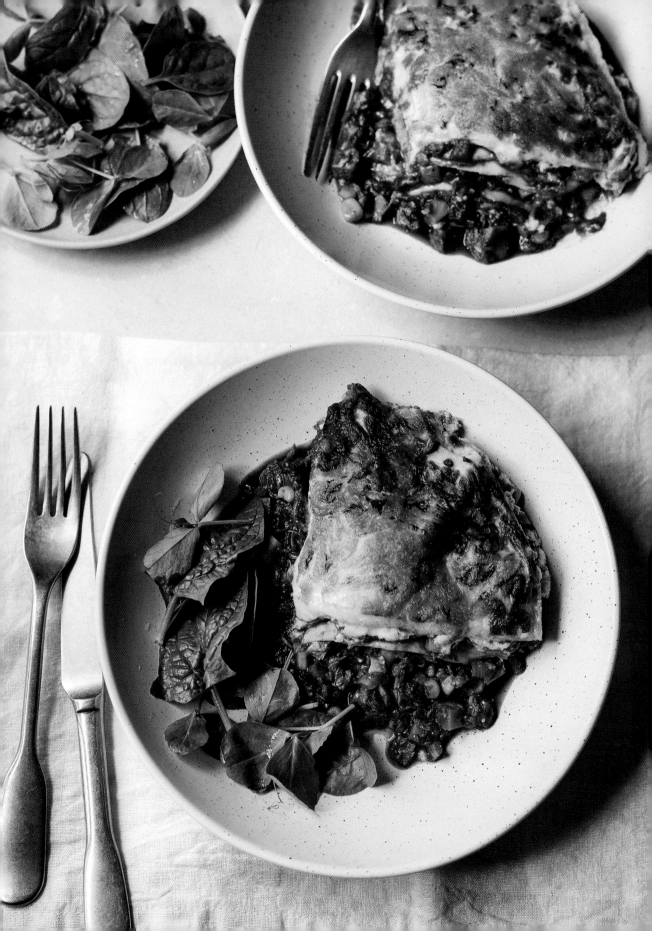

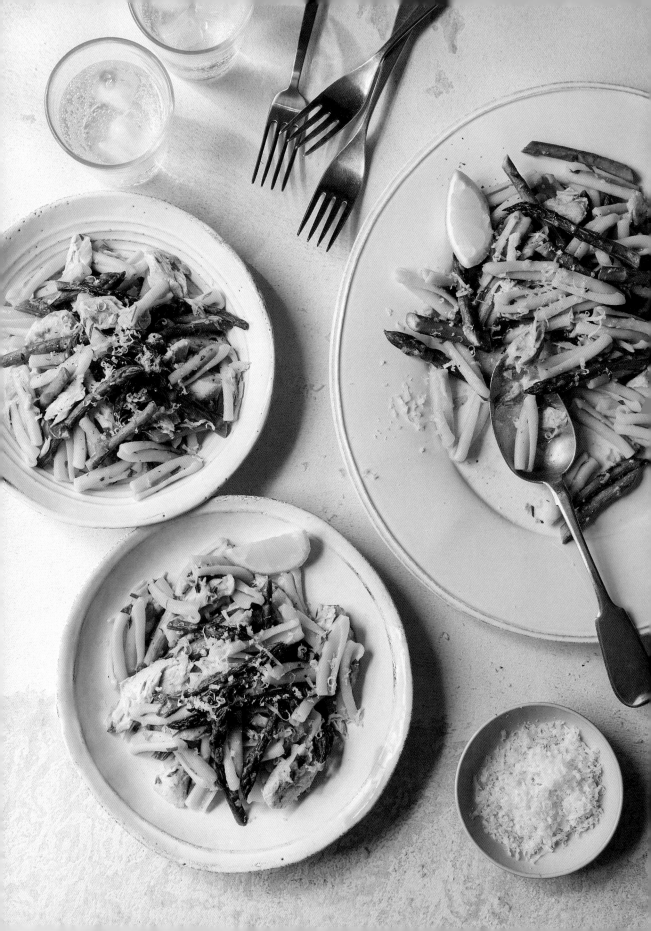

BUTTER SALMON AND ASPARAGUS PASTA

250g (9oz) dried
  casarecce pasta (or
  another similar pasta)
olive oil spray
350g (12½oz) salmon fillet
  (I use wild caught)
¼ tsp paprika
4 tsp butter
350g (12½oz) asparagus,
  trimmed and chopped
300g (10½oz) ripe fresh
  tomatoes, cored,
  deseeded and chopped
3 garlic cloves, crushed
60g (2oz) finely grated
  fresh Parmesan
2 tbsp finely chopped
  fresh parsley
2 tbsp fresh lemon juice
salt and freshly ground
  black pepper
lemon wedges, to serve

1. Cook the pasta according to the packet instructions until al dente. Reserve 60ml (4 tablespoons) of the pasta cooking water and set aside. Drain the pasta and spray with olive oil spray (this will prevent the pasta from sticking together). Toss to coat and set aside.

2. Preheat the air fryer to 200°C/400°F for 2 minutes.

3. Place the salmon directly in the air fryer basket or use a foil/silicone liner that fits. Push the salmon to one half of the air fryer basket, season the top with salt and pepper and add the paprika and half the butter to the top of the salmon.

4. Add the asparagus, tomatoes, garlic and a pinch of salt and pepper to the other half of the basket and dot with the remaining butter. Spray over the top with olive oil spray and air-fry for 7–9 minutes until the salmon and asparagus are cooked.

5. Remove the salmon from the air fryer, and flake into large pieces.

6. Add in the pasta and reserved pasta water, Parmesan, parsley and lemon juice and toss with the asparagus and tomatoes in the air fryer. Gently stir in the flakes of salmon and air-fry for a further minute or two to warm through.

7. Season to taste with freshly ground salt and black pepper. Serve with lemon wedges for additional flavour.

KCALS per serving 547   FAT 21.6g   SAT FAT 7.9g   CARBS 49.6g   SUGARS 5.4g   FIBRE 6.2g   PROTEIN 35.5g   SALT 0.44g

SERVES 4
PREP: **15 MINS**
COOK: **36 MINS**

CARIBBEAN PRAWN AND PINEAPPLE SKEWERS WITH COCONUT RICE

180g (6½oz) long-grain rice
olive oil spray
2 garlic cloves, crushed
1 tsp onion granules
pinch of dried thyme
100g (3½oz) canned
 black beans, drained
85g (3oz) canned sweetcorn
280ml (9½fl oz) hot
 chicken stock
200ml (7fl oz) coconut milk
400g (14oz) large prawns
 (shrimp), peeled
1 tbsp honey
½ small fresh pineapple,
 peeled, cored and
 sliced into chunks
1 red (bell) pepper, chopped
salt and freshly ground
 black pepper
2 spring onions
 (scallions), chopped
2 tbsp finely chopped
 fresh coriander/
 cilantro (optional)
squeeze of fresh lime juice

For the jerk seasoning
1 tbsp sweet paprika
1 tbsp garlic granules
1 tbsp onion granules
2 tsp salt
2 tsp cayenne pepper
½ tbsp allspice
2 tsp dried parsley

1. Preheat the air fryer to 200°C/400°F for 2 minutes.

2. Place a 20cm (8in.) cake barrel in the air fryer basket. Add in the rice and spray with olive oil spray. Turn to coat and air-fry for 1 minute until translucent.

3. Add in the garlic, onion granules, thyme, black beans, sweetcorn, stock and coconut milk with a pinch of salt and black pepper and stir to combine.

4. Cover tightly with foil and air-fry for 28 minutes, then remove the cake barrel and set it aside, leaving it tightly covered with the foil while you cook the prawn skewers. This will ensure the rice is cooked.

5. To make the jerk seasoning, mix all the ingredients in a bowl until well combined.

6. Add the prawns to a bowl with 1½ tablespoons of the jerk seasoning and the honey, reserving the rest of the seasoning for future use. Toss the prawns until well coated, then thread them onto metal skewers, alternating with the pineapple and red (bell) pepper pieces (see Note below). Spray all over with olive oil spray.

7. Preheat the air fryer to 190°C/375°F for 2 minutes.

8. Line the air fryer basket with non-stick baking paper or use the grill pan insert. Spray with olive oil spray. Add the prawn skewers and air-fry for 6–8 minutes until the prawns are cooked through. Turn the skewers halfway through cooking and spray with a little more olive oil spray.

9. Remove the foil from the rice and stir through the spring onion, coriander and a little squeeze of juice from a fresh lime. Serve the rice with the skewers.

KCALS per serving 448   FAT 10.9g   SAT FAT 7.8g   CARBS 63.7g   SUGARS 20.4g   FIBRE 7.1g   PROTEIN 20.2g   SALT 1.99g

1 tsp freshly ground
    black pepper
1 tsp dried thyme
½ tsp ground cumin
½ tsp ground nutmeg
½ tsp ground cinnamon
½ tsp ground ginger
pinch of red chilli flakes

Note

The number of skewers you use will depend on the size of both your skewers and your air fryer. I used 8 small ones (so 2 per person).

Quick swap

You can, if you prefer, use a branded jerk seasoning instead of making your own.

Tip

Store the unused 4½ tbsp of jerk seasoning in an airtight jar. You can also double or triple up the seasoning recipe to make a larger batch for future use.

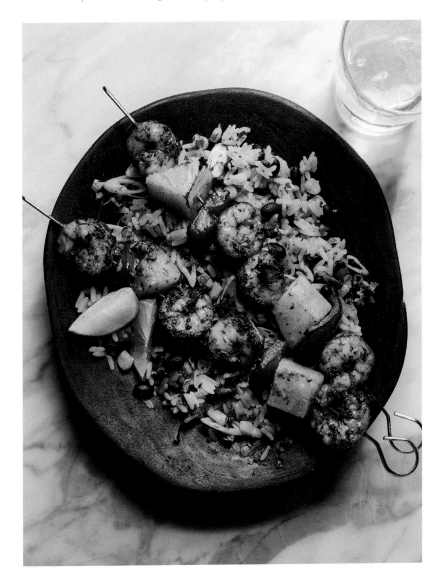

SWEET CHILLI SALMON BITES WITH SESAME GARLIC BROCCOLI

325g (11½oz) wild salmon fillets (skin removed), sliced into approx. 2.5cm (1in.) pieces

½ tsp sweet paprika

½ tsp garlic granules

½ tsp onion granules

¼ tsp cayenne pepper

¼ tsp ground ginger

salt and freshly ground black pepper

olive oil spray

250g (9oz) broccoli florets (or broccolini)

½ tbsp toasted sesame oil

1 garlic clove, finely chopped

1 tbsp soy sauce

3 tbsp sweet chilli sauce

To serve

1 spring onion (scallion), sliced

squeeze of lime juice

lime wedges

pinch of sesame seeds

1. Place the salmon in a bowl with the paprika, garlic granules, onion granules, cayenne pepper (if using), ginger and a pinch of salt and black pepper. Spray with olive oil spray and toss until evenly coated.

2. In another bowl, toss the broccoli in the sesame oil, garlic and soy sauce.

3. Preheat the air fryer at 200°C/400°F for 2 minutes.

4. Line the air fryer basket with non-stick baking paper and spray with olive oil spray. Arrange the salmon in one half of the basket and the broccoli in the other, then spray over the top with olive oil spray.

5. Air-fry for 5 minutes, turning the salmon and broccoli halfway through cooking.

6. Drizzle the sweet chilli sauce over the salmon, toss well to coat and cook for a further 1–2 minutes.

7. Transfer the salmon and broccoli to a serving plate. Sprinkle the sliced spring onion with a squeeze of lime juice over the salmon and a pinch of sesame seeds over the broccoli.

8. Serve with the lime wedges and enjoy!

Note

If you want to tone down the spiciness here, omit the cayenne pepper.

Side suggestions

Rice, noodles or (if you prefer a low-carb accompaniment) cauliflower rice.

Optional add-ons

For extra heat, sprinkle with some sliced red chilli.

KCALS per serving 447 FAT 25.9g SAT FAT 4.6g CARBS 8.4g SUGARS 5.2g FIBRE 6.1g PROTEIN 42g SALT 1.94g

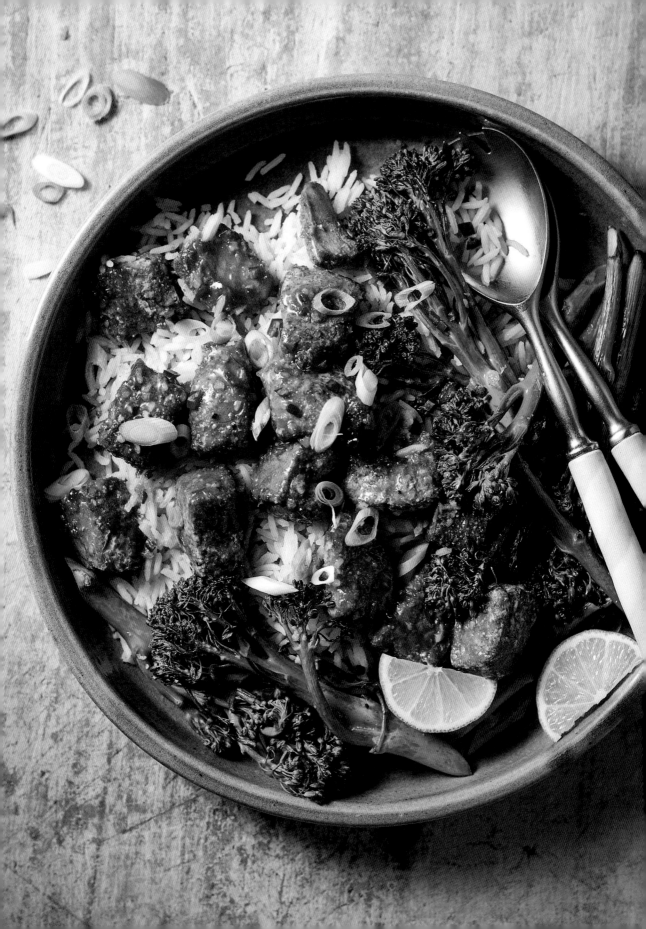

SERVES 4
PREP: **15 MINS**
COOK: **36 MINS**

125g (4½oz) courgettes
   (zucchini), halved
   lengthwise and diced
125g (4½oz) mushrooms,
   halved (or quartered
   if really big)
1 small onion, diced
80g (2¾oz) carrot,
   sliced into batons
1 tbsp butter, melted
1 tbsp soy sauce
olive oil spray
pinch of sesame seeds

For the yum yum sauce
4 tbsp fat-free Greek yogurt
2 tbsp light mayonnaise
2 tsp tomato ketchup
½ tbsp sweetener
½ tbsp mirin
1 tsp rice vinegar
½ tsp sweet paprika
½ tsp garlic granules
¼ tsp onion granules
1–2 tsp sriracha
   (optional for heat)

For the prawns
300g (10½oz) raw peeled
   large prawns (shrimp)
2 garlic cloves, minced
1½ tsp freshly grated ginger
1 tsp toasted sesame oil
1 tbsp hoisin sauce
1 tbsp soy sauce
freshly ground black pepper

HIBACHI PRAWNS WITH FRIED RICE

1. Cook the rice in advance (preferably the day before) and chill once cooked.

2. To make the yum yum sauce, whisk all the ingredients together in a jug along with a little water to loosen, and set aside.

3. Place the courgettes in a bowl. Add the mushrooms, onion and carrot with the butter and soy sauce and mix to combine.

4. Preheat the air fryer to 200°C/400°F for 3 minutes.

5. Place the vegetables directly into the air fryer basket or use a foil/silicone liner that fits. Spray with olive oil spray and air-fry for 4 minutes.

6. While the vegetables are cooking, place the prawns in a bowl. Add the garlic, ginger, toasted sesame oil, hoisin and soy sauces along with a pinch of black pepper and mix to combine.

7. When the vegetables have cooked for 4 minutes, push them to one side of the tray and add the prawns.

8. Spray over the top with olive oil spray, reduce the temperature to 190°C/375°F and air-fry the prawns and veg for a further 6–8 minutes until the prawns are cooked. Turn the prawns halfway through cooking.

9. While the prawns are cooking, prepare the rice. Place the cooked, chilled rice in a bowl. Add the garlic, ginger, sesame oil, soy sauces and spring onion and mix to combine. Season with a pinch of white pepper.

10. Transfer the prawn and vegetables to a plate and set aside. Spray the air fryer basket with olive oil spray and pour in the beaten egg. Cook at 190°C/375°F for a minute, then mix and cook for another 30 seconds until the egg is almost cooked.

KCALS per serving 384   FAT 10g   SAT FAT 3g   CARBS 52.1g   SUGARS 11.3g   FIBRE 2.9g   PROTEIN 20g   SALT 3.52g

For the rice

180g (6½oz) uncooked long- or medium-grain rice

2 garlic cloves, crushed

1½ tsp freshly grated ginger

1 tsp sesame oil

2 tbsp light soy sauce

1 tsp dark soy sauce

2 spring onions (scallions), chopped

1 egg, beaten

pinch of white pepper

11. Add in the rice to the egg and mix to combine, then spread out in the air fryer basket and spray over the top with olive oil spray and cook for 3 minutes. Stir, spread out again and cook for a further 2–3 minutes until completely heated through, then transfer to a bowl and cover with a plate to keep warm.

12. Return the veg and prawns to the air fryer for a minute or two to warm through.

13. Serve the prawns with the rice, sprinkled with a pinch of sesame seeds and serve the yum yum sauce on the side.

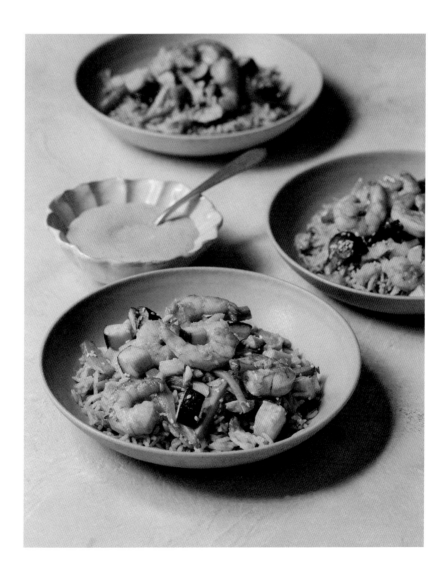

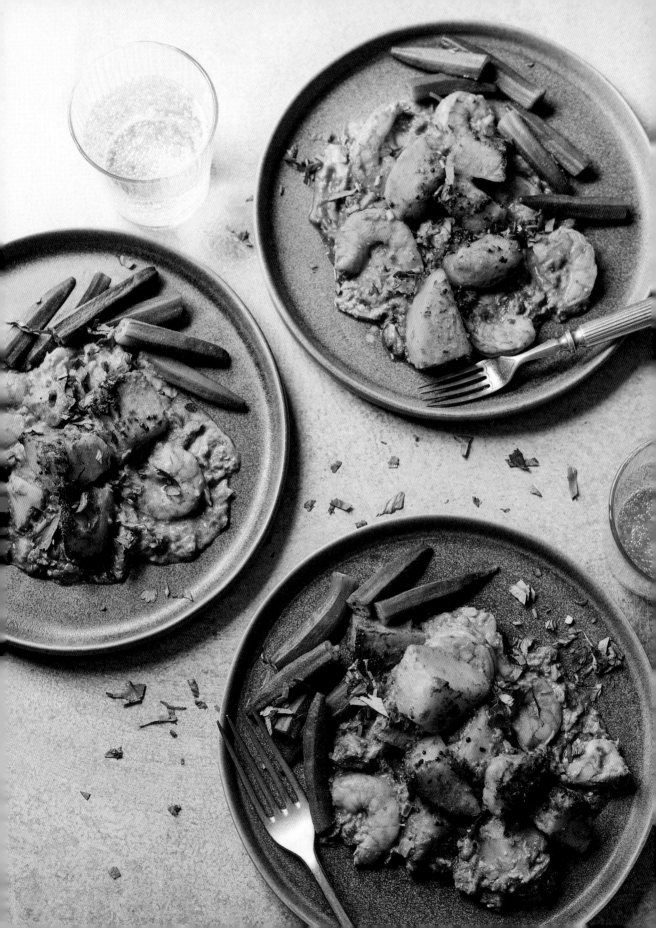

BOMBAY POTATO-TOPPED PRAWN AND FISH PIE

650g (23oz) yellow-fleshed potatoes, whole (skin on)
1 garlic clove, crushed
1 tsp grated fresh ginger
2 tsp curry powder
½ tsp black mustard seeds
salt

For the curry
olive oil spray
½ tbsp ghee
1 small onion, diced
¼ tsp fennel seeds, crushed
1½ tsp grated fresh ginger
3 garlic cloves, crushed
1½ tsp ground cumin
1½ tsp ground coriander
1 tsp hot chilli powder
1 tsp garam masala
¾ tsp ground turmeric
400g (14oz) good-quality canned plum tomatoes, crushed in a jug
2 tsp lemon juice
2 tsp sugar or sweetener
100ml (3½fl oz) hot chicken or fish stock
4 tbsp plain yogurt (don't use fat-free)
200g (7oz) firm white fish
200g (7oz) raw peeled large prawns (shrimp)
salt and freshly ground black pepper
finely chopped fresh coriander (cilantro), to serve

1. Pierce the potatoes and microwave for 6–8 minutes until fork tender but not really soft, then set aside to cool.

2. Preheat the air fryer to 200°C/400°F for 2 minutes.

3. To make the curry, place a foil (silicone) liner in the air fryer basket, and spray with olive oil spray. Add the ghee, onion and crushed fennel seeds and air-fry for 5 minutes.

4. Stir through the ginger, garlic, cumin, coriander, chilli powder, garam masala and turmeric, then add the tomatoes, lemon juice, sugar and stock. Air-fry for 8–10 minutes until the curry sauce is rich and thickened.

5. While the curry sauce is cooking, prepare the potatoes. Remove their skins and chop the flesh into 2.5cm (1in.) pieces. Place these in a bowl, then spray with olive oil and add the ginger, garlic, curry powder and black mustard seeds with a pinch of salt.

6. Once the curry sauce is ready, stir in the yogurt, add in the fish and prawns and gently stir to combine, ensuring they are covered in the sauce. Season to taste, then top with the potatoes and spray over the top with olive oil spray.

7. Reduce the temperature to 190°C/375°F and air-fry for 8–10 minutes until the potatoes are lightly golden at the edges and the fish and prawns are cooked. Sprinkle with fresh coriander and serve.

Side suggestions
Serve with a dollop of fat-free plain yogurt and some vegetables of your choice.

Optional add-ons
If you have some kasoori methi (fenugreek leaves), crush them and sprinkle them over the curry just before adding the potatoes for a punch of additional flavour.

Dairy free
Swap the ghee for vegetable oil and the plain yogurt for coconut milk.

KCALS per serving 316   FAT 5.8g   SAT FAT 2.2g   CARBS 36.8g   SUGARS 10.3g   FIBRE 6.3g   PROTEIN 26.1g   SALT 0.73g

olive oil spray
100g (3½oz) onion,
   thinly sliced
1 red (bell) pepper,
   thinly sliced
1 green (bell) pepper,
   thinly sliced
2 garlic cloves, crushed
pinch of salt
100ml (3½fl oz) hot
   chicken stock
30g (1oz) Cheddar, grated
50g (1¾oz) mozzarella, grated
pinch of red chilli flakes
4 wild caught salmon fillets
   (approx 180g/6½oz each)
1 tbsp honey

For the Fajita seasoning
1 tsp mild chilli powder
1 tsp sweet paprika
¾ tsp ground cumin
½ tsp garlic granules
½ tsp onion granules
pinch of cayenne pepper
   (if you like it more spicy)
salt and freshly ground
   black pepper

FAJITA STUFFED SALMON

1. Preheat the air fryer to 190°C/375°F for 3 minutes.

2. Line the air fryer basket with non-stick baking paper or use the grill pan insert. Spray with olive oil. Add the onion, (bell) peppers and garlic with a pinch of salt, then pour in the stock and mix to evenly distribute.

3. Spray over the top with olive oil spray and air-fry for 15 minutes until all the stock has evaporated and the peppers and onion are nice and softened/caramelized. Stir the vegetables halfway through cooking.

4. To make the fajita seasoning, mix all the ingredients in a bowl until well combined, then set aside.

5. Add the pepper and onion mixture to a bowl with the Cheddar, mozzarella and a pinch of chilli flakes. Mix until well combined.

6. Sprinkle the seasoning all over the salmon. Make a slit approximately three-quarters of the way into each salmon fillet to create a pocket and stuff with the pepper and cheese mixture. If the salmon fillet isn't deep enough, add the mixture to the top of the fillet.

7. Preheat the air fryer to 200°C/400°F for 2 minutes.

8. Add the salmon fillets to the air fryer basket, drizzle the salmon with the honey and spray over the top with olive oil spray.

9. Air-fry for 7–9 minutes until the salmon is cooked through and lovely and golden on top and the pepper and cheese stuffing is all melted.

Side suggestions

Salsa, soured cream, sliced avocado (or guacamole) and salad or seasoned rice.

KCALS per serving 490   FAT 29.4g   SAT FAT 7.8g   CARBS 9.1g   SUGARS 7.9g   FIBRE 3.2g   PROTEIN 45.6g   SALT 0.68g

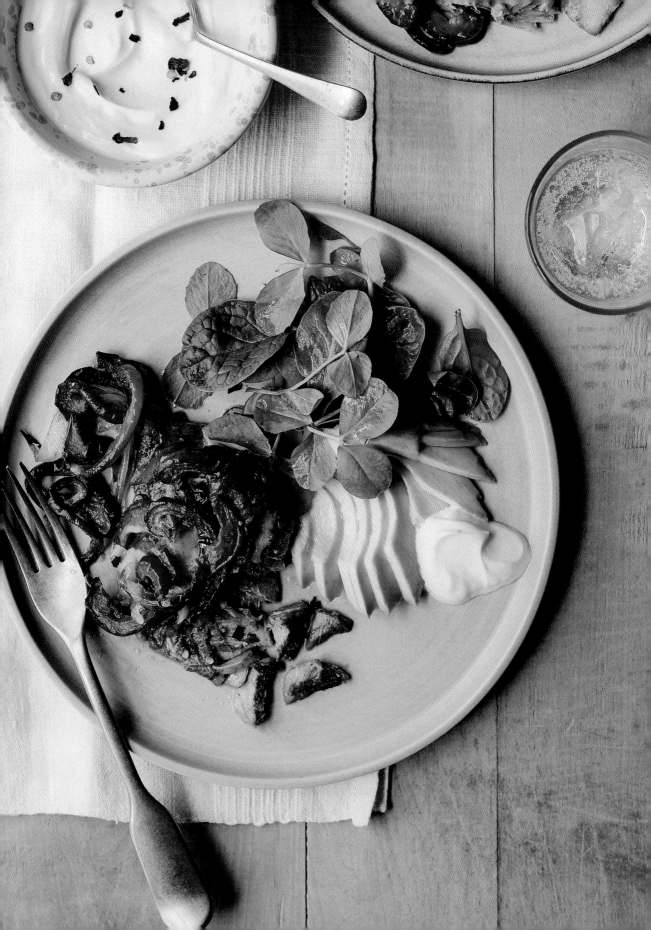

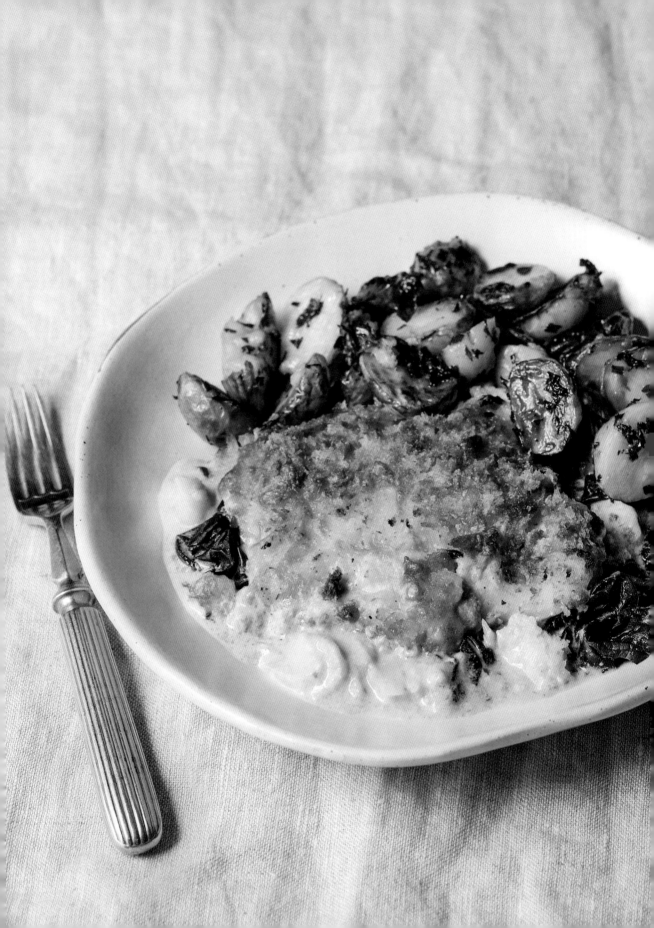

CHEESY, CREAMY COD GRATIN WITH HERBY CRUSHED POTATOES

350g (12½oz) baby potatoes (skin on), halved

2 garlic cloves, crushed

200ml (7fl oz) hot fish stock

olive oil spray

1½ tbsp finely chopped fresh parsley

1 tbsp finely chopped fresh chives

2 tsp butter

60g (2oz) spinach

250g (9oz) firm white fish fillets, e.g. tilapia or cod

60g (2oz) light cream cheese

1 tsp Dijon mustard

¼ tsp lemon zest

30g (1oz) mature Cheddar, grated

20g (¾oz) panko breadcrumbs

salt and freshly ground black pepper

1. Preheat the air fryer to 190°C/375°F for 2 minutes.

2. Place the potatoes in a 20cm (8in.) dish (it should be half the size of the air fryer basket) and place the dish in the air fryer. Add the garlic, 100ml (3½fl oz) stock and a pinch of salt. Toss to coat, then spray over the top with olive oil spray.

3. Air-fry for 15–18 minutes until the potatoes are tender. Turn halfway through cooking and spray again with olive oil spray. Squash down the cooked potatoes with a fork and mix through the parsley and chives.

4. Line the air fryer basket with non-stick baking paper or use the grill pan insert. Arrange the potatoes on one side of the basket and top with little knobs of the butter.

5. Place the spinach in a small dish that fills half the air fryer basket and top with the fish fillets. Season with salt and pepper.

6. In a jug, mix the cream cheese with the remaining 100ml (3½ fl oz) hot stock, along with the mustard and lemon zest and stir until melted. Pour this over the fish and spinach, pushing the fish down slightly into the sauce (the top of the fish fillets should be just above the sauce). Air-fry for 5 minutes.

7. While the fish and potatoes continue cooking, mix the Cheddar and panko in a bowl, rubbing them between your thumb and fingers until they are small crumbs.

8. Spread the breadcrumbs on top of the fish and cook for a further 6–7 minutes until the fish is cooked through and the topping is golden.

KCALS per serving 427   FAT 13.6g   SAT FAT 7.2g   CARBS 37.2g   SUGARS 4.8g   FIBRE 4.9g   PROTEIN 36.6g   SALT 1.43g

1 cauliflower head,
    broken into florets

1 tbsp olive oil

1 tsp mild chilli powder

2 garlic cloves, crushed

4 firm white fish fillets
    (approx 125g/4½oz each),
    sliced into large chunks
    (see Note below)

1 tbsp honey

¼ tsp smoked paprika

1 tsp sweet paprika

½ tsp onion granules

¼ tsp dried oregano

1 tsp ground cumin

salt and freshly ground
    black pepper

lime wedges, to serve

finely chopped fresh
    coriander, to serve

For the jalapeño crema

4 tbsp reduced-fat
    soured cream

2 tbsp light mayonnaise

1 small jalapeño, deseeded
    (leave the seeds in if
    you like a spicy sauce)

handful of finely chopped
    fresh coriander (cilantro)

1 tsp onion granules

1 garlic clove, crushed

1 tbsp fresh lime juice

pinch of salt and freshly
    ground black pepper

PERUVIAN SPICED FISH WITH CAULIFLOWER

1. To make the crema, blitz the ingredients in a mini blender until smooth. (Add a few drops of water to loosen if it is too thick to blend.) Taste and season well with salt and black pepper.

2. Place the cauliflower in a bowl, cover with boiling hot water and blanch for 4 minutes. Drain, then return to the bowl with half the olive oil, the chilli powder, 1 garlic clove, and a good pinch of salt and black pepper.

3. Place the cubed fish in another bowl with the honey, remaining garlic, smoked and sweet paprika, onion granules, oregano, cumin and a good pinch of salt and black pepper, along with the remaining olive oil. Toss to coat, then set aside.

4. Preheat the air fryer to 190°C/375°F for 2 minutes.

5. Add the cauliflower directly to the basket or line the air fryer basket with non-stick baking paper first and spray with olive oil spray. Air-fry for 5 minutes.

6. Move the cauliflower to one half of the basket, then add the cubed fish to the other half, spray with olive oil spray and air-fry for 10 minutes until the fish is cooked through.

7. Serve the fish and cauliflower with jalapeño crema, lime wedges and fresh coriander.

Side suggestions

This is delicious just as it is with the cauliflower,
or with rice or potatoes, or even as tacos.

Note

Tilapia or cod are fine here. Make sure the fish chunks are not too small.

KCALS per serving 237   FAT 9.1g   SAT FAT 1.5g   CARBS 11g   SUGARS 8g   FIBRE 3.8g   PROTEIN 26g   SALT 0.46g

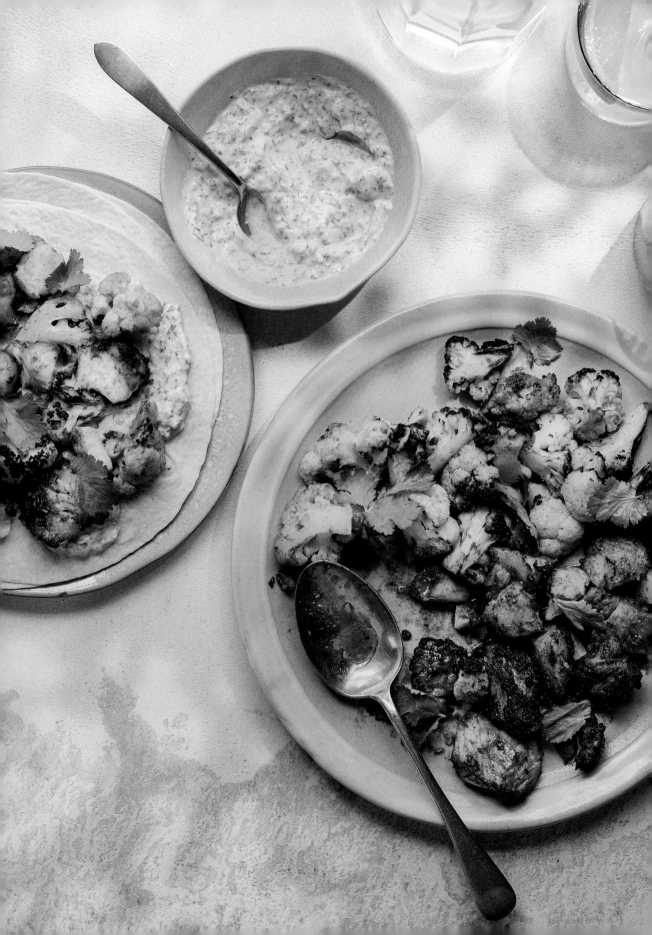

VEGETARIAN

BREAKFAST TORTILLA
PARCELS 165

FETA, VEGETABLE AND
RICE BAKE 167

GAMJI JORIM (KOREAN
BRAISED POTATOES) 168

SWEET POTATO AND
CHICKPEA CURRY 170

HALLOUMI FLATBREADS
WITH ROASTED VEG, HARISSA
SAUCE AND ROCKET 173

LOADED SRIRACHA FRIES 174

CAULIFLOWER KATSU CURRY 176

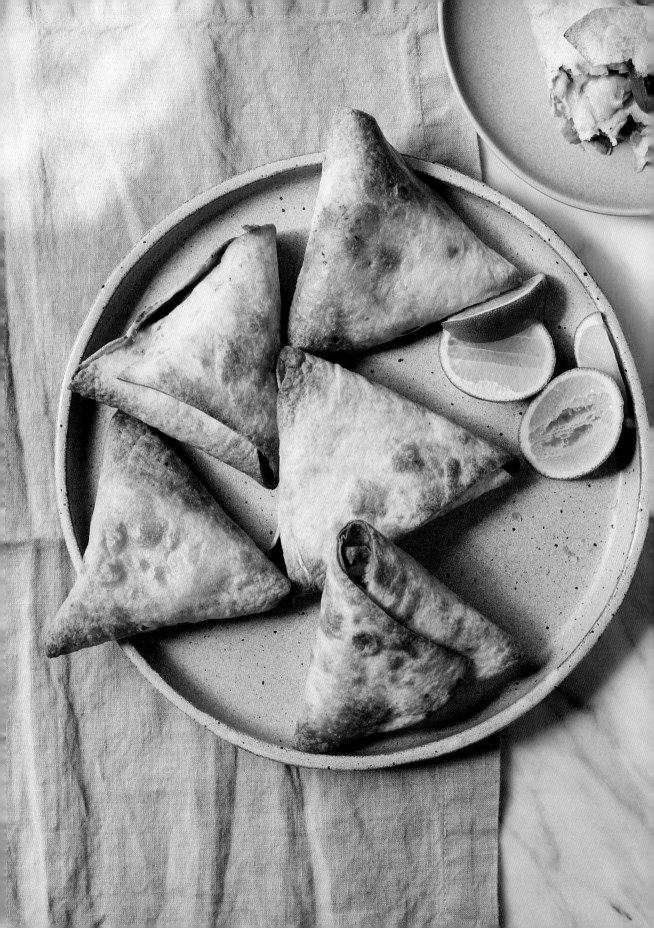

100g (3½oz) sweet potato, peeled and grated

200g (7oz) floury potatoes (skin on), whole

1 tsp sweet paprika

½ tsp onion granules

½ tsp garlic granules

olive oil spray

2 eggs, beaten

2 low-calorie white 20cm (8in.) tortilla wraps

65g (2¾oz) avocado, sliced

50g (2oz) Cheddar, grated

4 baby plum tomatoes, thinly sliced

salt and freshly ground black pepper

Optional add-ons

If you have some bagel seasoning, add a pinch to the top of the triangles once you've flipped them over to cook the other side, after spraying with more olive oil spray.

Not vegetarian?

Add in some cooked bacon, sausage or ham.

BREAKFAST TORTILLA PARCELS

1. Place the grated sweet potato in a bowl and set aside.

2. Microwave the potatoes in their skin for 4–5 minutes until slightly soft (not overcooked), then leave to cool slightly.

3. When cool enough to handle, remove the potato skins, and grate the potato into the bowl with the sweet potato. Add the paprika, onion granules, garlic granules and a pinch of salt and black pepper. Toss to coat.

4. Preheat the air fryer to 190°C/375°F for 2 minutes.

5. Line the air fryer basket with non-stick baking paper or use the grill pan insert. Spray with olive oil spray.

6. Add the grated potatoes. Flatten them out, spray over the top with olive oil spray and air-fry for 6–8 minutes until cooked. Stir the potatoes halfway through cooking, then flatten them out again and respray with olive oil spray.

7. Season the eggs with salt and black pepper and pour them into the potatoes, distributing them evenly so that they spread all over the bottom and cover the potatoes. Air-fry for 2–3 minutes until the eggs are just cooked. Slice into 8 equal-sized pieces.

8. Cut each tortilla wrap into half a circle, so you have 4 half circles. Fold a third of the tortilla over from the outer edge and then fold in the other third so you have a cone shape. Hold the cone flat in your hand and fill the tortilla with 2 potato slices, the avocado, cheese and tomato layers. Then, tuck in one side of the curved edge and fold over the other curved edge to seal (you should now have 4 triangular parcels). Place the parcels in the air fryer, seal-side down.

9. Spray over the top with olive oil spray and air-fry at 190°C/375°F for approximately 8 minutes, until lightly golden and crisp on the exterior. Turn the tortilla parcels halfway through cooking and spray with some more olive oil spray.

KCALS per serving 498   FAT 21.1g   SAT FAT 8.5g   CARBS 51.6g   SUGARS 7.9g   FIBRE 11g   PROTEIN 20.1g   SALT 0.96g

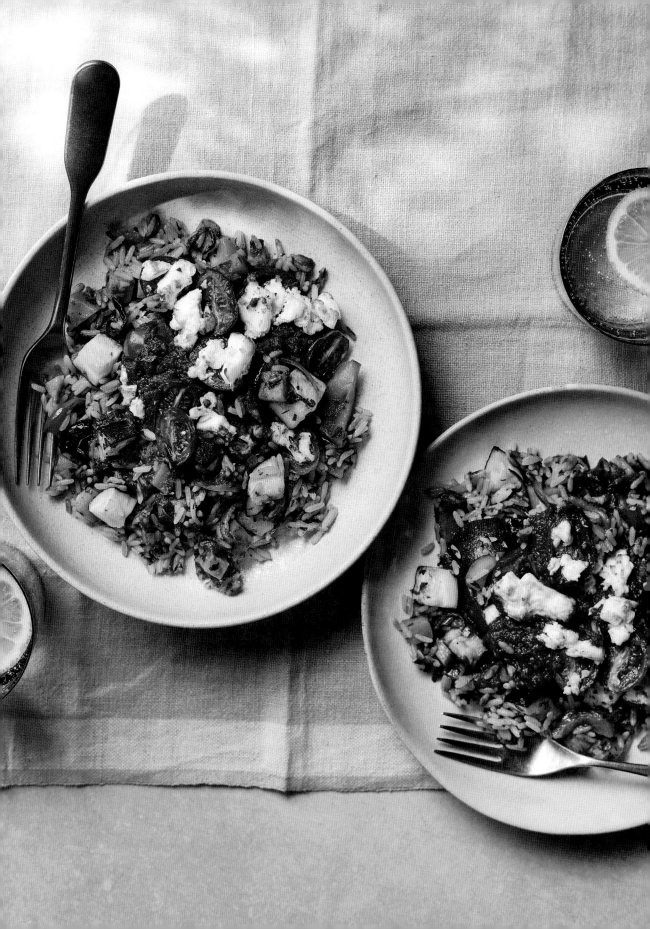

SERVES 4
PREP: 15 MINS
COOK: 30 MINS

olive oil spray

180g (6½oz) long-grain rice

475ml (16fl oz) hot
   vegetable stock

300g (10½oz) butternut
   squash, finely cubed

½ red (bell) pepper, diced

½ green (bell) pepper diced

150g (5¾oz) red onion,
   quartered and thinly sliced

1 tbsp extra virgin olive oil

2 garlic cloves, crushed

200g (7oz) courgettes
   (zucchini), chopped

200g (7oz) passata

2 tbsp tomato purée (paste)

200g (7oz) roasted
   red peppers in brine,
   well drained

1 tsp ground coriander

1 tsp garlic granules

1 tsp sweet paprika

½ tsp smoked paprika

½ tsp dried oregano

½ tsp red chilli flakes

2 tsp sugar or granulated
   sweetener

1 tbsp fresh lemon juice

2 tbsp finely chopped fresh
   coriander (cilantro) and
   parsley, plus extra to serve

16 baby plum
   tomatoes, halved

100g (3½oz) feta, crumbled

pinch of salt and freshly
   ground black pepper

FETA AND VEGETABLE RICE BAKE

1. Spray a saucepan with olive oil spray and fry the rice for a couple of minutes until translucent.

2. Add 475ml (16fl oz) vegetable stock. Bring to a boil, then reduce the heat and simmer just until the rice has absorbed stock, then cover and turn off the heat. Preheat the air fryer to 190°C/375°F for 2 minutes and leave the saucepan on the hob while you follow the next steps.

3. Add the butternut squash directly into the air fryer basket, along with the (bell) peppers, onion and olive oil and a good pinch of salt and black pepper and toss to coat. Air-fry for 10 minutes, shaking the basket halfway through cooking.

4. Add in the garlic and courgette and air-fry for a further 8–10 minutes, again shaking the basket halfway through cooking. Remove and set aside.

5. Blitz the passata, tomato purée and roasted red (bell) peppers a few times in a mini blender or food processor until smooth. Stir in all the seasonings with the sugar and add salt and pepper to taste, if necessary.

6. Mix the rice with the lemon juice, coriander and parsley. Season to taste with salt and black pepper, then stir in the roasted vegetables.

7. Place the rice in a 20cm (8in.) cake barrel and top with the tomato sauce. Lay the baby plum tomatoes on top, with the cut side facing upwards. Season the top of the tomatoes with a pinch of salt and black pepper and spray over the top with olive oil spray.

8. Air-fry at 200°C/400°F for 8–10 minutes until the tomatoes on top are lovely and roasted. Sprinkle with the feta and cook for a couple more minutes, until the cheese is lightly browned around the edges.

9. Serve sprinkled with some additional fresh parsley or coriander.

<u>Side suggestion</u>
*Serve with garlic yogurt. Mix 8 tbsp Greek yogurt with
1 crushed garlic clove. Add a pinch of salt and freshly ground
black pepper, 1 tsp dried parsley and a little lemon juice.*

KCALS per serving 393   FAT 10.3g   SAT FAT 4.1g   CARBS 58.6g   SUGARS 15.4g   FIBRE 8.2g   PROTEIN 12.4g   SALT 1.58g

GAMJI JORIM (KOREAN BRAISED POTATOES)

½ tbsp butter

½ tbsp oil of your choice

700g (1lb 9oz) baby potatoes (skin on), halved (leave whole if really small)

1 tsp sesame oil

For the braising sauce

3 tbsp soy sauce

2 tbsp maple syrup

2 garlic cloves, crushed

1 tbsp mirin

To serve

2 spring onions (scallions), chopped

pinch of sesame seeds

pinch of freshly ground black pepper

1. Preheat the air fryer to 190°C/375°F for 2 minutes.

2. Place the butter and oil directly into the air fryer basket, then add in the potatoes and air-fry for approximately 15–18 minutes until lightly golden and tender (not mushy). Shake the basket a few times while cooking as you want the potatoes to be lightly browned all over.

3. To make the braising sauce, pour all the ingredients into a bowl, add 2 tablespoons water and whisk to combine.

4. Once the potatoes are tender, add in the braising sauce, reduce the temperature to 185°C/360°F and air-fry for 3 minutes, then shake the basket and air-fry for another 2 minutes. The potatoes should all be coated in a lovely glaze.

5. Add the sesame oil and shake to coat.

6. Transfer the potatoes to a bowl and sprinkle with the chopped spring onion, a pinch of sesame seeds and a little black pepper.

Spicy variation

You can step up the spice in these potatoes by adding in a little gochujang or sriracha – 1–2 tsp max, as you don't want it to overpower the flavour of the braising liquid.

Tip

If you're using larger potatoes, I recommend peeling and dicing them into approx. 3cm (1¼in.) cubes. A waxy or semi-waxy variety is best as it will stay a little firmer – floury potatoes will go too mushy.

KCALS per serving 205   FAT 3.9g   SAT FAT 1.3g   CARBS 37.3g   SUGARS 11g   FIBRE 3.3g   PROTEIN 3.6g   SALT 1.6g

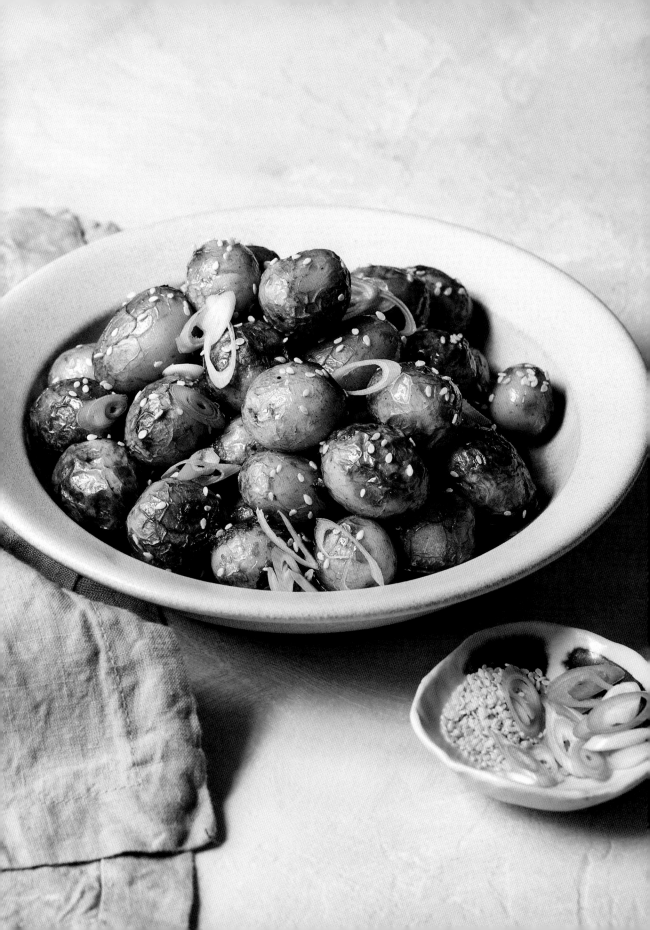

SWEET POTATO AND CHICKPEA CURRY

½ tbsp ghee or oil of
   your choice
400g (14oz) sweet potato,
   peeled and diced
100g (3½oz) red onion,
   quartered and sliced
400ml (14fl oz) can
   light coconut milk
400g (14oz) can
   chickpeas, drained
90g (3oz) fresh spinach,
   stems removed
salt
handful of chopped fresh
   coriander and sliced green
   chilli (optional), to serve

For the paste

2 tsp ground cumin
2 tsp ground coriander
2 tsp curry powder
1 tsp hot chilli powder
   (according to taste)
2 tbsp tomato purée (paste)
1 tbsp tamarind paste
1 tsp ground turmeric
3 garlic cloves, crushed
1 tbsp grated fresh ginger
2 tsp sugar
½ tsp salt

1. Place a 20cm (8in.) cake barrel in the air fryer basket. Add the ghee and preheat to 200°C/400°F for 2 minutes.

2. Add the sweet potato with a pinch of salt and air-fry for 15–18 minutes until the sweet potato is fork tender. Add the onion for the last 5 minutes of cooking.

3. To make the paste, blitz all the ingredients along with 60ml (4 tablespoons) water in a mini food processor.

4. Add the paste to the sweet potato and onion, stir to combine and air-fry for 2 minutes.

5. Pour in the coconut milk and chickpeas and stir. Air-fry for 13 minutes.

6. Add the spinach, stir to combine and cook for a further minute, until just wilted. Taste and season with salt as needed.

7. Serve sprinkled with coriander and fresh sliced green chilli (if you like).

KCALS per serving 326   FAT 12.7g   SAT FAT 7.8g   CARBS 39.4g   SUGARS 13.1g   FIBRE 9.6g   PROTEIN 8.6g   SALT 0.9g

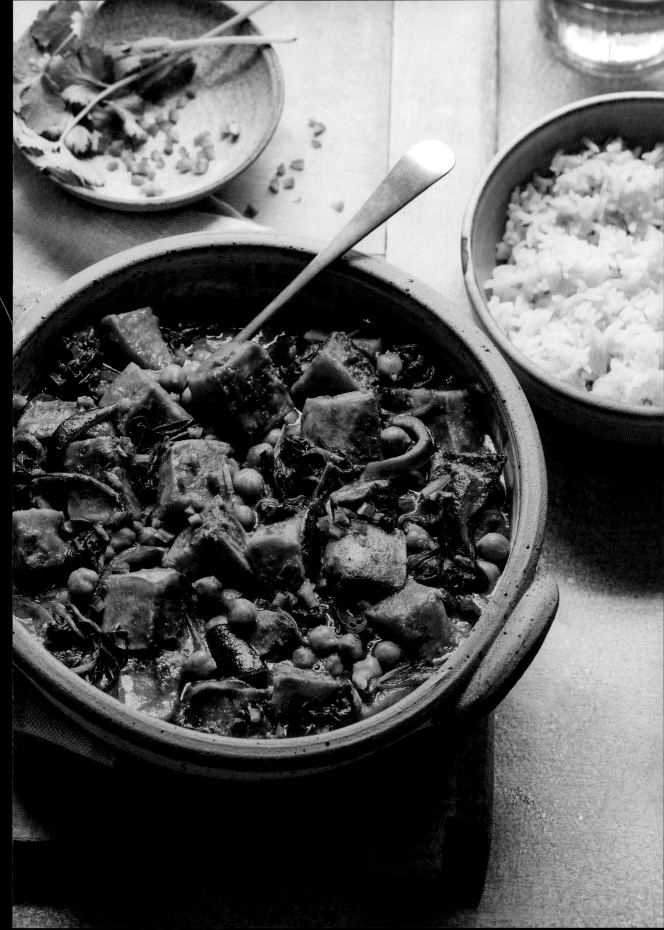

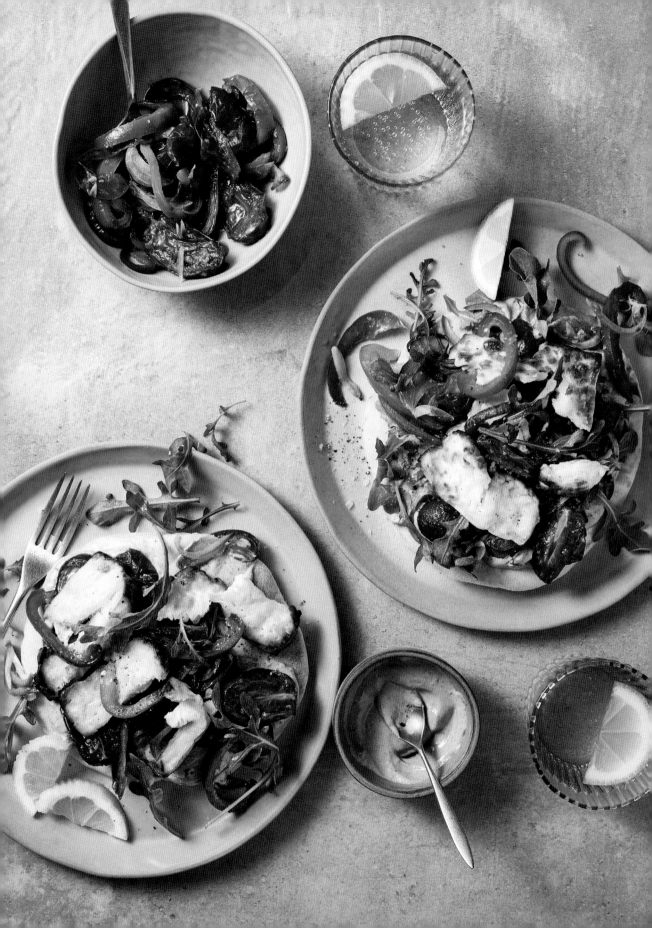

SERVES 4
PREP: **15 MINS**
COOK: **25 MINS**

HALLOUMI FLATBREADS WITH ROASTED VEG, HARISSA SAUCE AND ROCKET

1 red (bell) pepper,
    thinly sliced

1 green (bell) pepper,
    thinly sliced

20 baby plum
    tomatoes, halved

1 small red onion, halved
    and thinly sliced

2 garlic cloves, minced

olive oil spray

½ tbsp maple syrup

½ tbsp red wine vinegar

250g (9oz) halloumi
    cheese, sliced

4 handfuls of rocket (arugula)

1 tsp lemon juice

salt and freshly ground
    black pepper

For the harissa sauce

1 tbsp harissa paste (see Note)

1 tbsp light mayonnaise

3 tbsp plain fat-free yogurt

To serve

4 low-calorie flatbread thins
    (or pitta/naan), warmed

salt and freshly ground
    black pepper

½ small red onion, thinly sliced

1. Preheat the air fryer to 200°C/400°F for 2 minutes.

2. Place the (bell) peppers, tomato, onion and garlic directly into the air fryer basket. Spray with olive oil spray and air-fry for 10 minutes until the vegetables are softened.

3. Add the maple syrup and red wine vinegar, mix everything together and air-fry for a further 2 minutes. Remove and set aside.

4. Add the halloumi, spray again and air-fry at 190°C/375°F for 10 minutes. Turn the halloumi for the last 3 minutes of cooking.

5. To make the harissa sauce, whisk the harissa with the mayonnaise and yogurt in a jug until well combined.

6. Place the rocket in a bowl. Spray with some olive oil spray, sprinkle over the lemon juice and season with a pinch of salt and black pepper. Toss to coat.

7. Once the halloumi is cooked you can warm the flatbread.

8. If you want to reheat the vegetables, just heat them for a minute or so in the air fryer at 200°C/400°F.

9. Spread the warmed flatbreads with the harissa sauce and top with the rocket, vegetables and halloumi.

Note
If you're not keen on spicy food, halve the amount of harissa.

KCALS per serving 488   FAT 18.4g   SAT FAT 10.8g   CARBS 51.6g   SUGARS 13g   FIBRE 5.4g   PROTEIN 26.5g   SALT 2.77g

SERVES 4
PREP: 15 MINS
COOK: 40 MINS

LOADED SRIRACHA FRIES

1kg (2lb 4oz) potatoes, peeled and sliced into fries

80g (2¾oz) Chinese leaf cabbage, shredded

1 red (bell) pepper, finely diced

60g (2oz) onion, finely diced

½ tsp chilli powder

1 tsp sweet paprika

2 tsp cooking oil of your choice

2 garlic cloves, chopped

salt and freshly ground black pepper

60g (2oz) grated Cheddar, to serve

2 spring onions (scallions), sliced, and sesame seeds, to serve

For the fries
½ tsp sweet paprika

½ tsp onion granules

½ tsp garlic granules

salt

olive oil spray

For the sriracha mayo
2 tbsp light mayonnaise

1 tbsp plain fat-free yogurt

2 tsp sriracha

1. Soak the potatoes in ice-cold water for at least 45 minutes! Rinse and pat dry.

2. Preheat the air fryer to 190°C/375°F for 2 minutes.

3. Place the cabbage and red (bell) pepper directly into the air fryer basket. Add the onion, chilli powder, paprika, salt and black pepper and oil. Toss to mix, then air-fry for 8–10 minutes until the vegetables are tender. Add the garlic and shake the basket halfway through cooking. Remove the vegetables and set aside.

4. To prepare the fries, add the paprika, garlic granules, onion granules and salt to the potatoes and toss to coat. Spray a few times with olive oil spray.

5. Preheat the air fryer to 200°C/400°F and cook the potatoes for 22–25 minutes. Toss a couple of times in the basket throughout cooking. Transfer to a warmed plate.

6. To make the sriracha mayo, whisk the mayonnaise with the yogurt in a bowl, then add the sriracha. Add a little water if necessary to loosen it slightly for drizzling.

7. Reheat the cabbage mixture for a couple of minutes and place it on top of the fries. Top with the grated Cheddar, drizzle all over with sriracha mayo and sprinkle with sliced spring onion and sesame seeds.

Tip

For perfect cut fries, invest in a potato chipper. I have had mine for years and love it.

You can increase the sriracha to your desired taste if you wish to add more heat to the sriracha mayo.

KCALS per serving 291 FAT 9.7g SAT FAT 3.6g CARBS 38.4g SUGARS 6.3g FIBRE 5.9g PROTEIN 9.7g SALT 0.52g

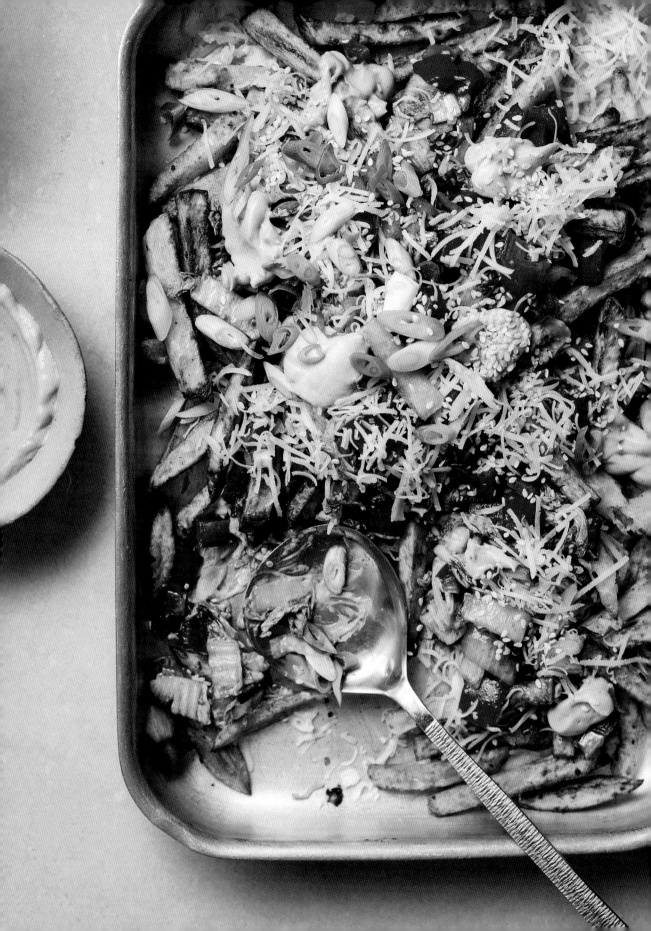

SERVES 2
PREP: **15 MINS**
COOK: **35 MINS**

50g (1¾oz) panko
   breadcrumbs
½ tbsp toasted sesame seeds
1 tsp sweet paprika
½ tsp onion granules
½ tsp garlic granules
350g (12oz) small
   cauliflower florets
1 large egg, beaten
salt and freshly ground
   black pepper
90g (3½oz) jasmine rice
pinch of black sesame seeds

For the katsu sauce
1 onion (100g/3½oz),
   finely diced
150g (5½oz) butternut
   squash, grated
olive oil spray
2 garlic cloves, crushed
1 tsp finely grated fresh ginger
2 tbsp curry powder
pinch of cayenne
   pepper (optional)
200ml (7fl oz) light
   coconut milk
240ml (8½fl oz) hot
   vegetable stock
1 tbsp soy sauce
½ tbsp maple syrup or honey

For the salad
30g (1oz) shredded carrot
50g (1¾oz) cucumber ribbons
handful of finely chopped
   fresh coriander (cilantro)

CAULIFLOWER KATSU CURRY

1. Place a 20cm (8in.) cake barrel in the air fryer basket.

2. Preheat the air fryer to 190°C/375°F for 2 minutes.

3. To make the sauce, place the onion and butternut squash into the cake barrel and spray with olive oil spray. Air-fry for 7 minutes until the vegetables are softened. Turn a few times to ensure they don't burn.

4. Add the garlic, ginger, curry powder and cayenne, if using, and air-fry for a minute.

5. Whisk the coconut milk, stock, soy sauce and maple syrup in a jug until well combined. Pour this into the cake barrel with the onion and butternut squash and air-fry for 10 minutes.

6. Transfer the mixture to a blender and blitz until the sauce is really smooth (if it's too thick, just add in a little stock or water).

7. While the sauce is cooking, you can prep the cauliflower. Mix the panko, toasted sesame seeds and seasonings on a flat plate until all combined. Dip the cauliflower florets in the beaten egg, then roll in the panko breadcrumb mixture to coat all over.

8. Preheat the air fryer to 190°C/375°F for 2 minutes.

9. Cook the jasmine rice according to the packet instructions.

10. While the rice is cooking, you can air-fry the cauliflower. Line the air fryer basket with non-stick paper. Add the cauliflower florets (ensuring there is a space between each one), spray over the top with olive oil spray and air-fry for 15–17 minutes until golden and cooked through. Turn halfway through cooking and spray again with olive oil spray. Remove and set aside.

11. Add the katsu sauce to the air fryer for a minute or two, just to reheat.

12. Arrange the cauliflower on a plate and spoon over the sauce. Top the rice with a pinch of black sesame seeds and serve alongside a salad of carrot, cucumber and coriander.

KCALS per serving 578   FAT 15.5g   SAT FAT 7.8g   CARBS 83.6g   SUGARS 19.2g   FIBRE 12.4g   PROTEIN 19.8g   SALT 1.99g

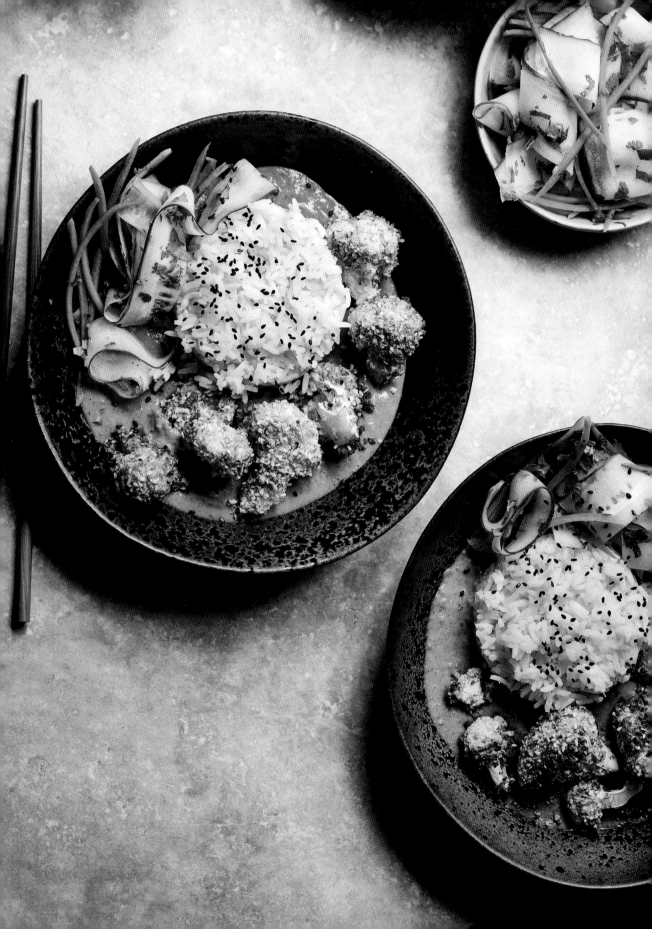

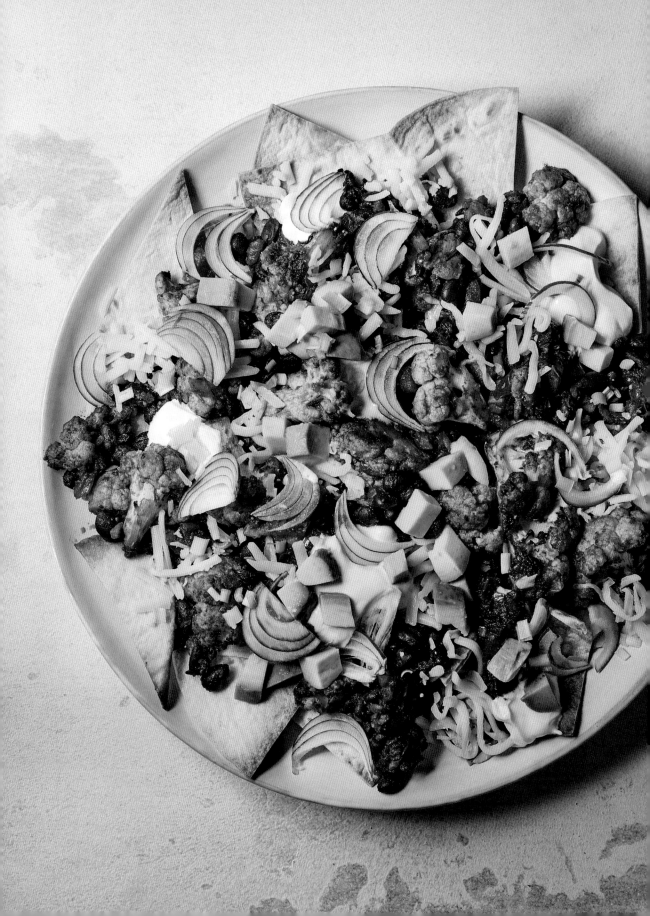

SERVES 2
PREP: 15 MINS
COOK: 21 MINS

2 x 20cm (8in.) low-calorie
  tortilla wraps, cut into
  triangles (white are best)
olive oil spray
300g (10½oz)
  cauliflower florets
1½ tsp sweet paprika
1 tsp mild chilli powder
½ tsp ground cumin
½ tsp onion granules
½ tsp garlic granules
salt and freshly ground
  black pepper
150g (5½oz) canned
  black beans, drained
120g (4oz) mild or medium
  shop-bought salsa
20g (¾oz) Cheddar, grated
20g (¾oz) mozzarella, grated
1 spring onion (scallion), diced
½ red onion, thinly sliced
65g (2½oz) avocado, diced
4 tbsp reduced-fat
  soured cream

CAULIFLOWER AND BLACK BEAN NACHOS

1. Toss the tortilla triangles with salt.

2. Preheat the air fryer basket to 190°C/375°F for 2 minutes. Spray the air fryer basket with olive oil spray, add the tortilla traingles, then spray over the top with more olive oil and air-fry for 6 minutes. Turn halfway through cooking and spray again until lightly golden and crisp. Remove the tortilla chips and set aside.

3. Blanch the cauliflower in boiling hot water for 3 minutes, then drain and pat dry.

4. Preheat the air fryer to 190°C/375°F for 2 minutes.

5. Transfer the cauliflower to a bowl and spray all over with olive oil spray. Add the seasonings, toss to coat and spray again.

6. Place the cauliflower in the air fryer basket and cook for 10 minutes. Turn the cauliflower halfway through cooking and respray with olive oil spray.

7. Mix the beans with the salsa in a bowl until well combined. Scatter the salsa bean mix in between the roasted cauliflower in the air fryer basket and cook for a further 5 minutes. Transfer to a large plate.

8. Add the tortilla triangles back to the basket for a minute, just to reheat them, then spread them out on a large plate. Scatter with the roasted cauliflower and black beans and sprinkle with the Cheddar, mozzarella, spring onion, red onion and avocado. Dollop the soured cream randomly over the top and serve.

Swaps

If you prefer, you can skip the tortillas and serve with cooked rice in bowls. Equally delicious!

KCALS per serving 495 FAT 18g SAT FAT 7.2g CARBS 52.9g SUGARS 12.3g FIBRE 18g PROTEIN 21.4g SALT 0.89g

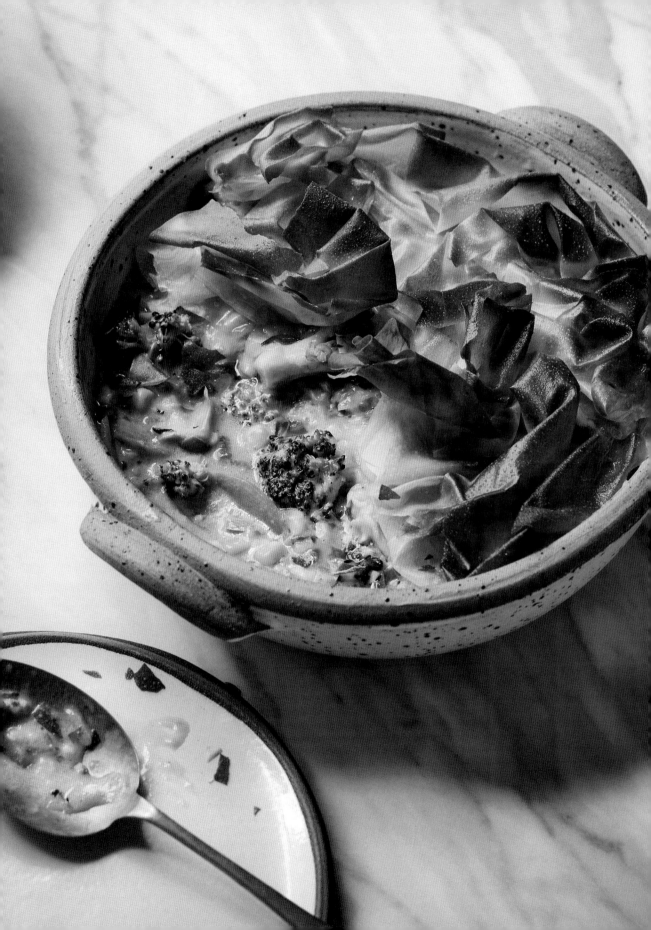

1 tbsp butter

1 onion, diced

3 garlic cloves, crushed

80g (2¾oz) carrot,
thinly sliced

1 red (bell) pepper,
finely diced

1 green (bell) pepper,
finely diced

200g (7oz) broccoli florets

salt and freshly ground
black pepper

100g (3½oz) frozen or
canned sweetcorn

salt and freshly ground
black pepper

200ml (7fl oz) hot
vegetable stock

200ml (7fl oz) semi-
skimmed milk

1½ tbsp cornflour (cornstarch)

100g (3½oz) mature
Cheddar, grated

4 sheets of filo pastry

olive oil spray

1 egg, beaten

RAINBOW VEGETABLE PIE

1. Place a 20cm (8in.) cake barrel or ovenproof dish into the air fryer basket and add the butter.

2. Preheat the air fryer to 190°C/375°F for 2 minutes.

3. Place the onion in the cake barrel, along with the garlic, carrot, (bell) peppers and broccoli. Add a pinch of salt and black pepper and air-fry for 7 minutes.

4. Add the sweetcorn and pour in the hot stock. Whisk the milk with the cornflour and add this too, stirring to combine.

5. Air-fry for 5 minutes, uncovered, then cover tightly with foil and air-fry for a further 15 minutes, until the sauce has thickened.

6. Remove the foil and sprinkle the Cheddar over the vegetables.

7. Spray the filo pastry sheets with olive oil spray, then roughly screw them up into balls and place on top of the pie filling. Brush the top with beaten egg and air-fry at 185°C/360°F for 12–15 minutes, until golden on top.

Tip

If you prefer your broccoli more tender, parboil it until tender and add at step 4.

Swaps

If you prefer, you can swap the filo for reduced-fat puff pastry – just enough to cover the top of the pie. It will need to be cooked at 200°C/400°F for approximately 10 minutes.

KCALS per serving 346 FAT 15.8g SAT FAT 8.5g CARBS 31.8g SUGARS 12g FIBRE 7.2g PROTEIN 15.7g SALT 0.97g

SERVES 4
PREP: 15 MINS
COOK: 25 MINS

250g (9oz) dried pasta
  bows (farfalle)
olive oil spray
200g (7oz) courgettes
  (zucchini), halved and sliced
200g (7oz) cherry
  tomatoes, halved
1 small onion, thinly sliced
½ red (bell) pepper, sliced
½ yellow (bell) pepper, sliced
4 garlic cloves, crushed
1 tsp herbes de Provence
80g (2¾oz) frozen or
  canned sweetcorn
salt and freshly ground
  black pepper
1 tbsp finely chopped
  fresh basil
1 tbsp finely chopped
  fresh parsley

For the lemon sauce
1 tbsp extra virgin olive oil
1 tbsp fresh lemon juice
30g (1oz) vegetarian
  Italian-style hard cheese
salt and freshly ground
  black pepper

PASTA PRIMAVERA

1. Cook the pasta according to the packet instructions until al dente. Reserve 80ml (2¾fl oz) of the pasta cooking water and set aside. Drain the pasta and spray with olive oil spray (this will prevent the pasta from sticking together). Toss to coat and set aside.

2. Preheat the air fryer to 190°C/375°F for 2 minutes.

3. Place all the vegetables (except the sweetcorn), with the herbes de Provence and a good pinch of salt and black pepper, into the air fryer basket or use a foil/silicone liner that fits. Spray the vegetables all over with olive oil spray and air-fry for 6 minutes.

4. Turn the vegetables, add the sweetcorn and spray again all over with olive oil spray. Air-fry for a further 5–6 minutes.

5. While the vegetables are cooking, make the sauce. Whisk together the olive oil and lemon juice in a small bowl. Add the vegetarian Italian-style hard cheese and a pinch of salt and pepper. Slowly add in the reserved hot pasta water and whisk again until everything is well combined.

6. Once the vegetables are cooked, add the pasta to the air fryer. Toss the pasta in the sauce with the basil and parsley and air-fry for 2 minutes. Season as needed with a pinch of salt and black pepper.

Optional add-ons
Sprinkle in some pine nuts at step 6 before air-frying for the last 2 minutes.

KCALS per serving 338   FAT 7.3g   SAT FAT 2.2g   CARBS 51.9g   SUGARS 6.9g   FIBRE 6.4g   PROTEIN 12.8g   SALT 0.13g

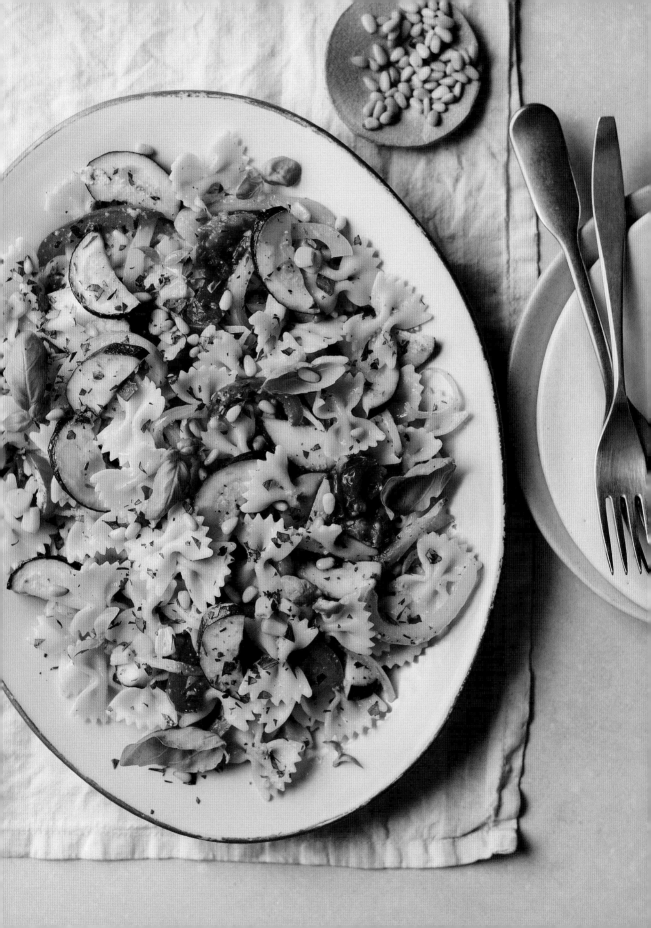

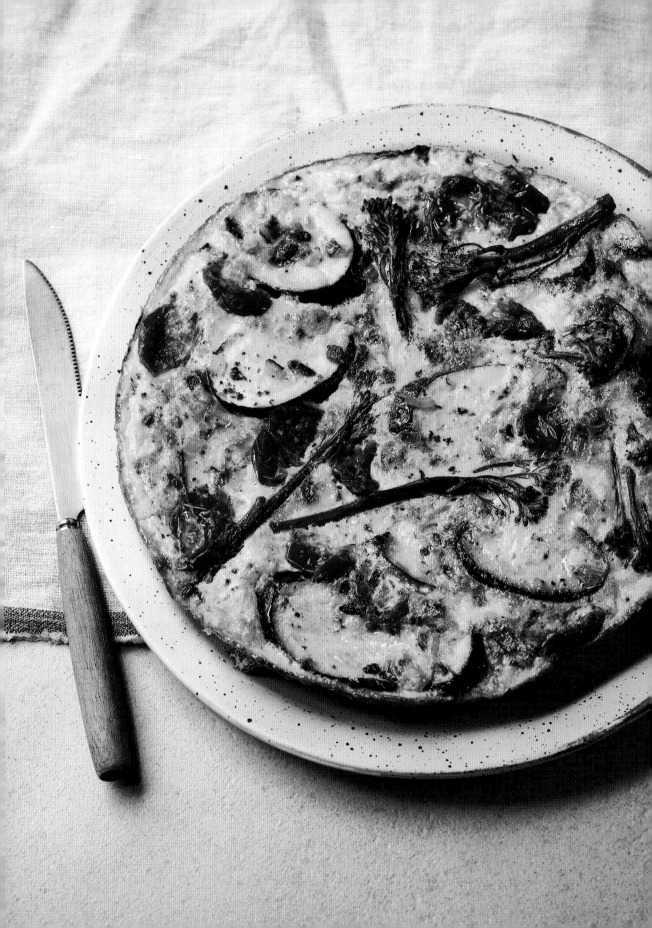

BROCCOLI, COURGETTE AND SUN-DRIED TOMATO FRITTATA

1 small onion, finely diced

160g (5¾oz) courgettes (zucchini), halved lengthways and sliced

olive oil spray

160g (5¾oz) broccoli florets

60g (2oz) sun-dried tomatoes in oil, drained and chopped

2 garlic cloves, crushed

pinch of chilli flakes

7 large eggs

2 tbsp semi-skimmed milk

60g (2oz) Cheddar, grated

salt and freshly ground black pepper

1. Preheat the air fryer to 200°C/400°F for 2 minutes.

2. Place the onion and courgettes in the air fryer basket. Add a pinch of salt and black pepper and spray with olive oil spray. Air-fry for 2 minutes.

3. Add the broccoli, sun-dried tomatoes, garlic and chilli flakes, stir to combine, spray with olive oil spray and air-fry for 5 minutes.

4. Blitz the eggs, milk and Cheddar in a blender until smooth.

5. Line a 20cm (8in.) cake barrel with non-stick baking paper and pour in the egg mixture. Add the vegetables and mix to distribute.

6. Place the cake barrel in the air fryer and air-fry at 160°C/325°F for 20 minutes until the mixture is set and golden. After 10 minutes, tightly cover the top with foil so that it doesn't go too brown.

7. Leave to rest for 10 minutes, then slice and enjoy.

Not vegetarian?

Add some cooked chicken or cooked bacon before air frying the egg mixture at step 6.

KCALS per serving 286   FAT 16.5g   SAT FAT 6.3g   CARBS 9.3g   SUGARS 7.7g   FIBRE 4.2g   PROTEIN 22.8g   SALT 0.82g

ROASTED TOMATO AND WHITE BEAN GNOCCHI

1 small onion (approx. 80g/2¾oz), finely diced

2 garlic cloves, crushed

455g (1lb) good-quality ripe fresh tomatoes, halved

1 tsp herbes de Provence

1 tbsp extra virgin olive oil

1 tbsp tomato purée (paste)

1 tbsp white wine vinegar

1 tbsp maple syrup

olive oil spray

handful of fresh basil leaves

500g (1lb 2oz) gnocchi (fresh or vacuum-packed is fine)

400g (14oz) can white beans (navy, haricot or cannellini), drained

30g (1oz) Italian-style vegetarian hard cheese or Cheddar, grated

100g (3½oz) mozzarella, torn into pieces

salt and freshly ground black pepper

1. Preheat the air fryer to 190°C/375°F for 3 minutes.

2. Place the onion and garlic directly into the air fryer basket or use a foil/silicone liner that fits.

3. Season the cut side of the tomatoes with salt and black pepper and place them, cut-side down, on top of the onion and garlic. Season over the top with another pinch of salt and black pepper and sprinkle with the herbes de Provence.

4. Drizzle the olive oil all over the top and air-fry for 15 minutes.

5. Stir the tomato purée, white wine vinegar and maple syrup into the mixture, spray over the top with olive oil spray and air-fry for a further 5 minutes.

6. Transfer everything in the air fryer to a blender with a couple of fresh basil leaves (reserve some to serve) and blitz until smooth.

7. Add the sauce back to the air fryer basket with the gnocchi and air-fry for 8–10 minutes at 190°C/375°F. Stir in the beans, top with the vegetarian Italian-style hard cheese and mozzarella and air-fry for a further 8 minutes at 180°C/350°F until melted and golden.

8. Serve scattered with some additional basil leaves.

Swap
If you prefer, use granulated sweetener instead of the maple syrup.

Not vegetarian?
You can swap the beans for some cooked sausage, chicken, bacon or mini meatballs.

Tip
Make up some batches of this sauce and freeze it so you have a quick and easy healthy pasta sauce whenever you need it.

KCALS per serving 431   FAT 11.4g   SAT FAT 5.6g   CARBS 61.1g   SUGARS 9.3g   FIBRE 9g   PROTEIN 16.4g   SALT 0.8g

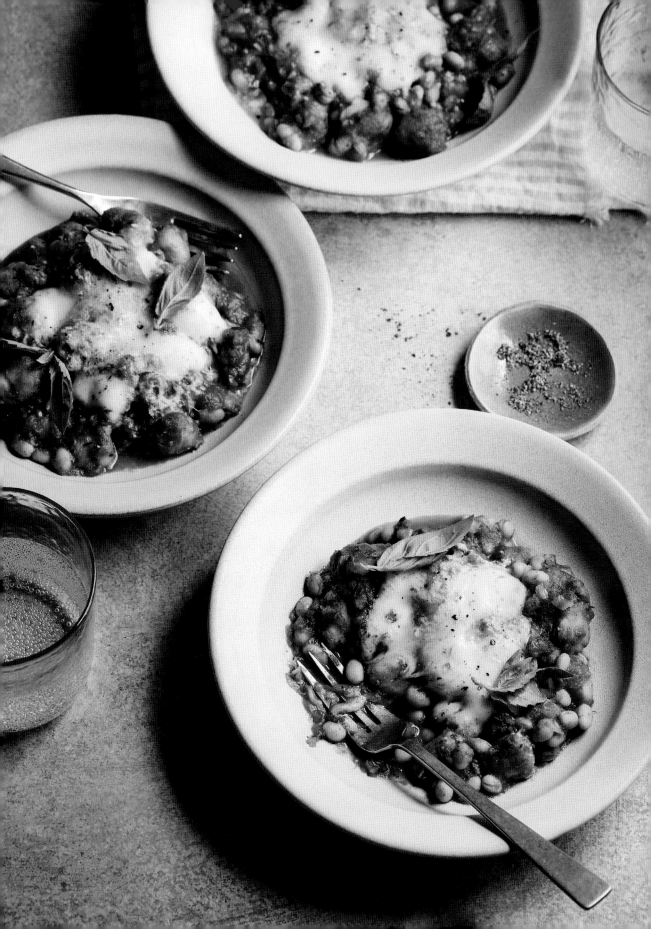

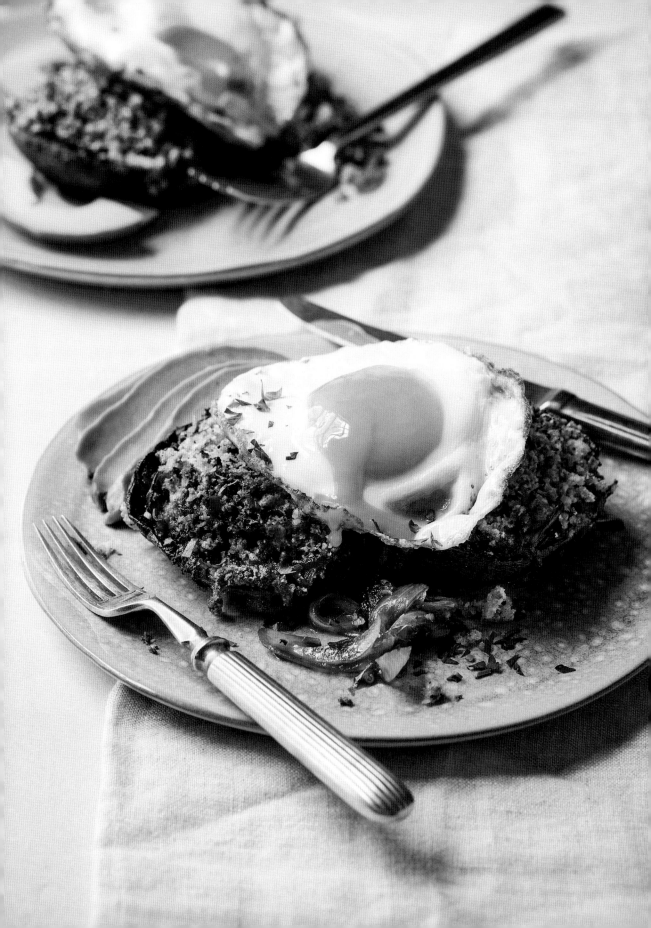

SERVES 2
PREP: 15 MINS
COOK: 25 MINS

30g (1oz) panko breadcrumbs
60g (2oz) Cheddar,
    finely grated
1 tsp dried parsley
½ tsp garlic granules
½ tsp onion granules
4 large portobello mushroom
    caps (approx 80g/2¾oz)
2 tsp Marmite
olive oil spray
200g (7oz) onions, thinly
    sliced (I use a mixture
    of white and red)
2 garlic cloves, crushed
½ tbsp butter, melted
1 tbsp honey
½ tsp red chilli flakes
salt and freshly ground
    black pepper

CHEESY MARMITE STUFFED MUSHROOMS

1. Mix together the panko, Cheddar, parsley, onion and garlic granules in a bowl and rub between your thumb and fingers to create small crumbs.

2. Remove and discard the gills from the mushrooms. Remove the stems and roughly chop Set the mushrooms aside.

3. Preheat the air fryer to 200°C/400°F for 2 minutes.

4. Dissolve the Marmite in 100ml (3½fl oz) hot water and set aside.

5. Spray the air fryer basket with olive oil spray or use a foil/silicone liner that fits and spray that. Add the sliced onion, mushroom stems and garlic to the air fryer. Pour in the butter and the Marmite liquid and stir to combine. Air-fry for 10 minutes.

6. Add the honey, red chilli flakes and mix to combine, then spray over the top with olive oil spray and cook for a further 5 minutes until the onions are caramelized and the liquid has pretty much evaporated. Remove and set aside.

7. Reduce the air fryer temperature to 180°C/350°F. Add the mushrooms, cap-side facing upwards to the grill pan insert and spray with olive oil spray. Air-fry for 5 minutes.

8. Turn the mushrooms and spray with olive oil spray. Fill with the caramelized Marmite onions, top with the Cheddar breadcrumb mixture and air-fry for a further 8–10 minutes until the topping is all golden.

Serving suggestions

These mushrooms are delicious just as they are, or served with a fried or poached egg and avocado.

KCALS per serving 329   FAT 16.3g   SAT FAT 8.7g   CARBS 30g   SUGARS 15.7g   FIBRE 4.9g   PROTEIN 13.2g   SALT 1.54g

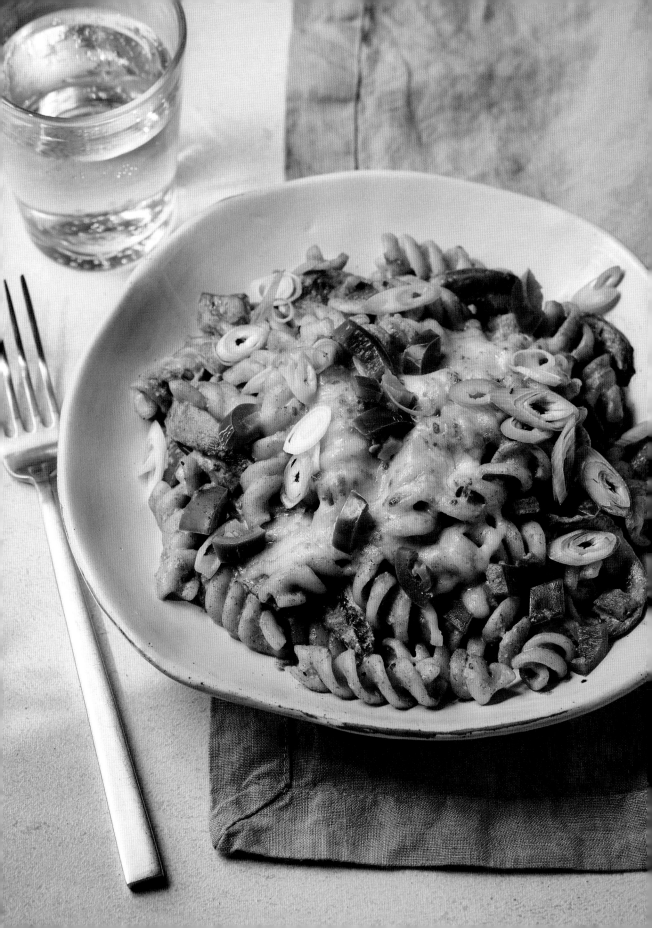

SERVES 4
PREP: 10 MINS
COOK: 23 MINS

300g (10½oz) dried
   fusilli pasta

olive oil spray

80g (2¾oz) onion,
   finely diced

1 green (bell) pepper,
   finely diced

200g (7oz) ripe tomatoes,
   cored, deseeded
   and finely diced

150g (5½oz)
   mushrooms, sliced

1 tbsp sweet paprika

1 tsp mild chilli powder

1 tsp onion granules

1 tsp garlic granules

½ tsp ground cumin

½ tsp freshly ground
   black pepper

pinch of salt

5½ tbsp hot vegetable stock

1 tbsp white wine vinegar

150g (5½oz) light
   cream cheese

80ml (2¾fl oz) semi-
   skimmed milk

1 tbsp maple syrup

60g (2oz) Cheddar, grated

50g (1¾oz) mozzarella, grated

3 spring onions (scallions),
   thinly sliced

2 tbsp pickled jalapeños
   (approx 30g/1oz)

TEXAN-STYLE VEGGIE FUSILLI

1. Cook the pasta according to the packet instructions until al dente. Reserve 60ml (4 tablespoons) of the pasta cooking water and set aside. Drain the pasta and spray with olive oil spray (this will prevent the pasta from sticking together). Toss to coat and set aside.

2. While the pasta is cooking, place the onion, green (bell) pepper and tomatoes directly into the air fryer basket and spray with olive oil spray. Toss to coat and air-fry for 5 minutes at 190°C/375°F.

3. Add the mushrooms, seasonings, stock and white wine vinegar and stir to combine. Make a space in the centre, then add the cream cheese and spray over the top with olive oil spray. Air-fry for 12 minutes at 180°C/350°F.

4. Add in the milk, pasta, maple syrup and reserved pasta water and toss to coat. Air-fry for approximately 2 minutes, until the pasta is all coated in a creamy sauce. Sprinkle the grated Cheddar and mozzarella over the top, then the spring onion and pickled jalapeños. Air-fry for a few more minutes until melted and lightly golden.

Swap
If you prefer, use granulated sweetener instead of the maple syrup.

Not vegetarian?
Add in some cooked bacon or chicken.

Optional add-on
The pickled jalapeños on top already add a nice warmth to the pasta but, if you like extra heat, you can add in a pinch of cayenne.

KCALS per serving 477 FAT 12g SAT FAT 6.4g CARBS 65.6g SUGARS 12.1g FIBRE 7.6g PROTEIN 22.9g SALT 1.01g

SERVES 4
PREP: 15 MINS
COOK: 30 MINS

½ white onion, finely diced

½ red onion, finely diced

½ green (bell) pepper, finely diced

½ red (bell) pepper, finely diced

75g (2½oz) carrot, very finely diced

150g (5½oz) butternut squash, finely diced

1 tbsp sweet paprika

1 tbsp extra virgin olive oil

olive oil spray

3 garlic cloves, crushed

½ tsp fennel seeds, crushed

1 tsp Italian herb seasoning

pinch of red chilli flakes

500ml (18fl oz) hot vegetable stock

400g (14oz) can chopped tomatoes

400g (14oz) can green or brown lentils, drained

couple of dashes of Tabasco sauce (optional)

1 tbsp maple syrup

2 tbsp finely chopped fresh parsley

salt and freshly ground black pepper

LENTIL CASSEROLE

1. Preheat the air fryer to 190°C/375°F for 2 minutes.

2. Place the onions, (bell) peppers, carrot, butternut squash and paprika with a good pinch of salt and black pepper to the air fryer basket, drizzle with the olive oil, toss to coat and air-fry for 10 minutes. Stir halfway through cooking and spray with some olive oil spray to prevent burning.

3. Add in the garlic, fennel, mixed herbs, red chilli flakes and about 50ml (3 tablespoons) of the stock. Stir to coat and air-fry for 5 minutes, until the vegetables are tender.

4. Transfer the vegetables to a 20cm (8in.) cake barrel and add in the tomatoes and lentils. Stir in the remaining stock with the Tabasco (if using) and maple syrup. Air-fry for 15 minutes.

5. Stir in the parsley, taste and season with more salt and pepper as needed.

Side suggestions

This is delicious with air-fried potatoes or delicious low-calorie mashed potatoes.

Cover 700g (1lb 9oz) chopped peeled potatoes and 2 garlic cloves with 1 litre (33¾fl oz) vegetable or chicken stock, and bring to a simmer for 15–20 minutes until fork tender. Drain (but reserve the stock), mash until smooth, using some of the reserved stock if needed, then stir in 4 tbsp reduced-fat soured cream until creamy and 1 tbsp chopped chives. Season to taste with salt and black pepper and (if you don't mind a few extra calories), add 1 tbsp butter to the top and let it melt all over the mash.

Not vegetarian?

Add in some cooked shredded chicken for the last 5 minutes of cooking.

KCALS per serving 185   FAT 4.4g   SAT FAT 0.6g   CARBS 24.4g   SUGARS 14.5g   FIBRE 8.6g   PROTEIN 7.5g   SALT 0.37g

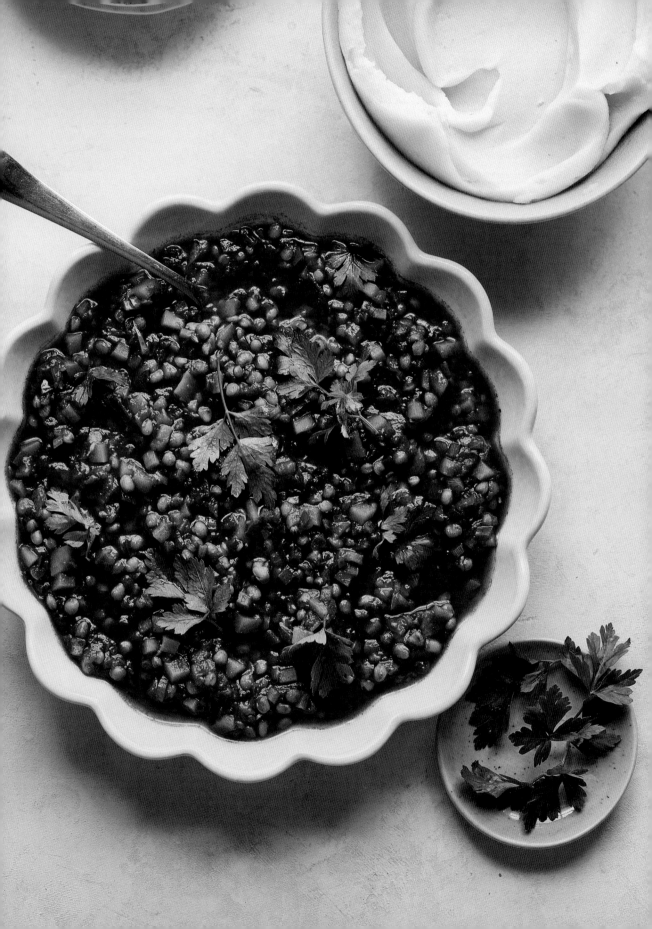

SWEET TREATS

CINNAMON SUGAR TWISTS WITH
DARK CHOCOLATE DRIZZLE 199

AIR-FRIED OREOS 200

PEACH AND RASPBERRY
STREUSEL CUSTARD TOASTS 203

ORANGE, CRANBERRY AND
WHITE CHOCOLATE SCONES 205

BISCOFF TORTILLA CANNOLI
WITH RASPBERRIES 206

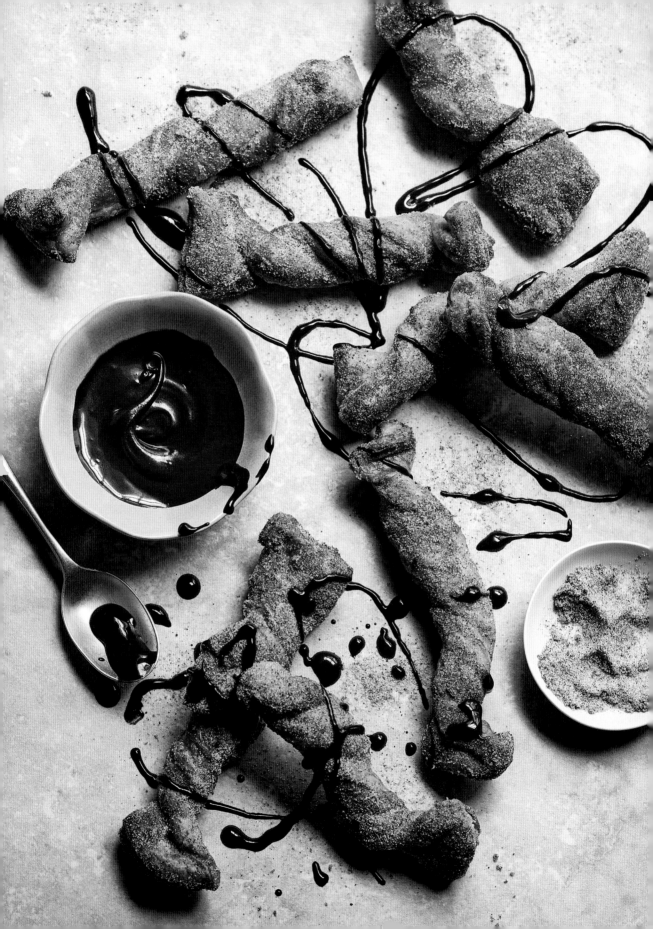

MAKES 8 TWISTS
PREP: 10 MINS
COOK: 10 MINS

CINNAMON SUGAR TWISTS WITH DARK CHOCOLATE DRIZZLE

120g (4¼oz) ready-rolled sheet of reduced-fat puff pastry
olive oil spray
2 tsp sugar
¼ tsp ground cinnamon
15g (½oz) dark chocolate

1. Preheat the air fryer to 190°C/375°F for 2 minutes.

2. Slice the puff pastry into 8 equal-sized strips and twist each one a few times.

3. Line the air fryer basket with non-stick baking paper or use the grill pan insert. Spray with olive oil spray. Add the pastry twists and air-fry for 8–10 minutes until golden. Turn the twists halfway through cooking and spray again.

4. Place the twists in a bowl and spray with olive oil spray. Turn, then sprinkle over the sugar and cinnamon and toss to coat. Spread the twists out on a flat plate or board.

5. Melt the dark chocolate in a microwave at 10-second intervals and drizzle over the twists.

KCALS per serving 67   FAT 3.5g   SAT FAT 1.8g   CARBS 7.7g   SUGARS 1.8g   FIBRE 0.4g   PROTEIN 1g   SALT 0.12g

160g (5¾oz) self-raising
flour (plus a little
extra for dusting)
180g (6½oz) fat-free
vanilla Greek yogurt
olive oil spray
8 oreos
dusting of icing sugar
(approx. 1 tsp)

AIR-FRIED
OREOS

1. Place the flour and yogurt in a bowl and mix with a wooden spoon or silicone spatula until it all comes together in a ball (do not mix with your hands).

2. Dust a clean surface with some additional flour and lightly dust the top of the dough, then knead a couple of times until you have a large, flattened ball. Divide into 8 equal-sized pieces.

3. Grease the air fryer basket with olive oil spray (or line the basket with sprayed non-stick baking paper).

4. Roll one of the 8 pieces of dough into a rough oval shape. Place an oreo on half of the oval and fold over the unfilled side. Shape into a rough circle to seal the dough and carefully place in the air fryer. Repeat with the other 7 pieces of dough.

5. Preheat the air fryer to 190°C/375°F for 2 minutes.

6. Mist the doughed oreos with spray oil, then transfer to the air fryer basket (make sure you leave a small space around each one as they will rise slightly).

7. Cook in the air fryer for approximately 5 minutes until golden on top, then carefully turn and cook the other side for 2 minutes.

8. Transfer to a plate or rack and allow to cool slightly, then dust with icing sugar and serve.

KCALS per serving 142   FAT 2.7g   SAT FAT 0.7g   CARBS 24.1g   SUGARS 5.6g   FIBRE 1.1g   PROTEIN 4.8g   SALT 0.27g

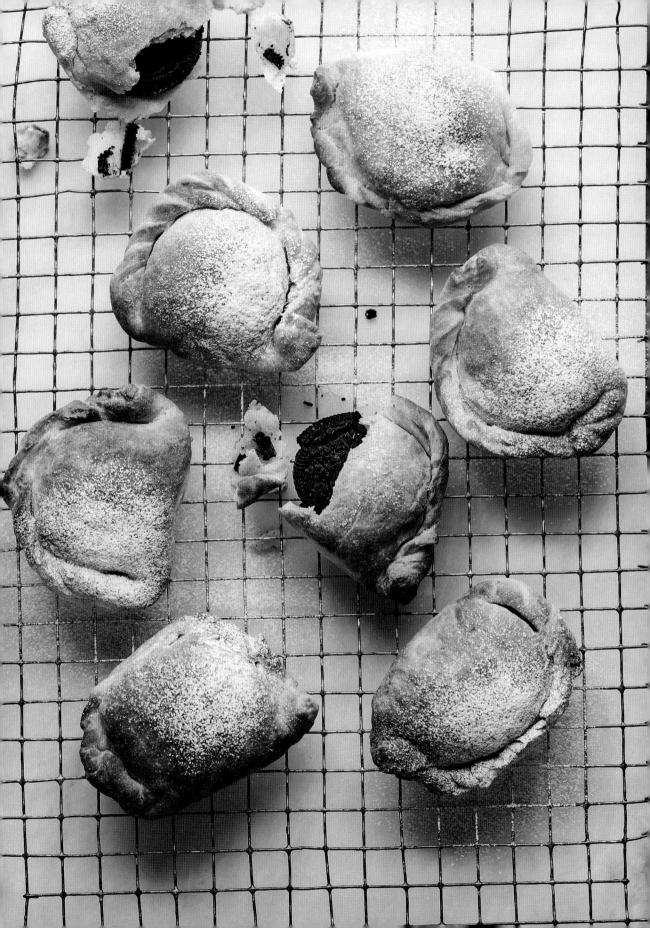

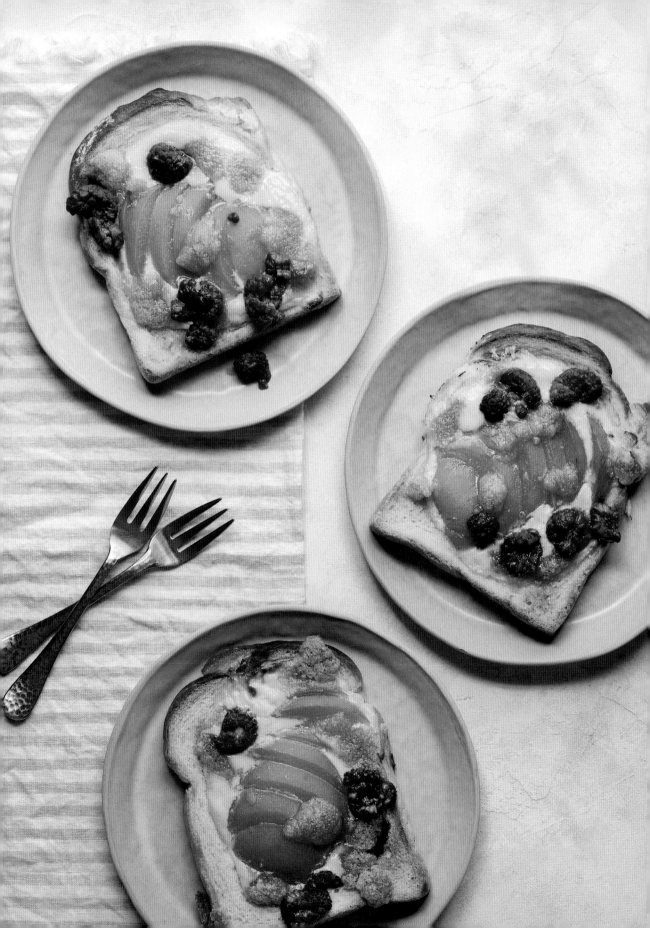

PEACH AND RASPBERRY STREUSEL CUSTARD TOASTS

3 slices of low-calorie bread of
    your choice (white is best)
olive oil spray
1 egg
70g (2½oz) fat-free
    Greek yogurt
2 tsp maple syrup or honey
120g (4¼oz) canned peaches
12 raspberries
½ tbsp brown granulated
    sweetener
6g Demerara sugar
2 tsp plain flour
1 tsp unsalted butter

1. Preheat the air fryer to 190°C/375°F for 2 minutes.

2. Using a spoon, make a dip in the middle of each bread slice, just up to the crust.

3. Line the air fryer basket with non-stick baking paper or use the grill pan insert. Spray with olive oil spray. Add the bread, with the dip facing downwards, and cook for about a minute, until it feels slightly firmer but is not browned.

4. Whisk the egg with the Greek yogurt and maple syrup in a bowl, then spoon this into the dips in the bread.

5. Add the peach slices, along with the raspberries, to each slice of bread.

6. Mix the sugar, flour and butter in a bowl until it is well combined, but be careful not to overmix (the mixture should be slightly clumpy). Scatter this over the top.

7. Place the slices back in the air fryer and air-fry for 5–6 minutes until the custard is set and the toast and streusel topping are lightly golden.

<u>Variations</u>
You can use any fruit for this.

KCALS per serving 163   FAT 3.9g   SAT FAT 1.5g   CARBS 23g   SUGARS 10.9g   FIBRE 2.6g   PROTEIN 7.8g   SALT 0.31g

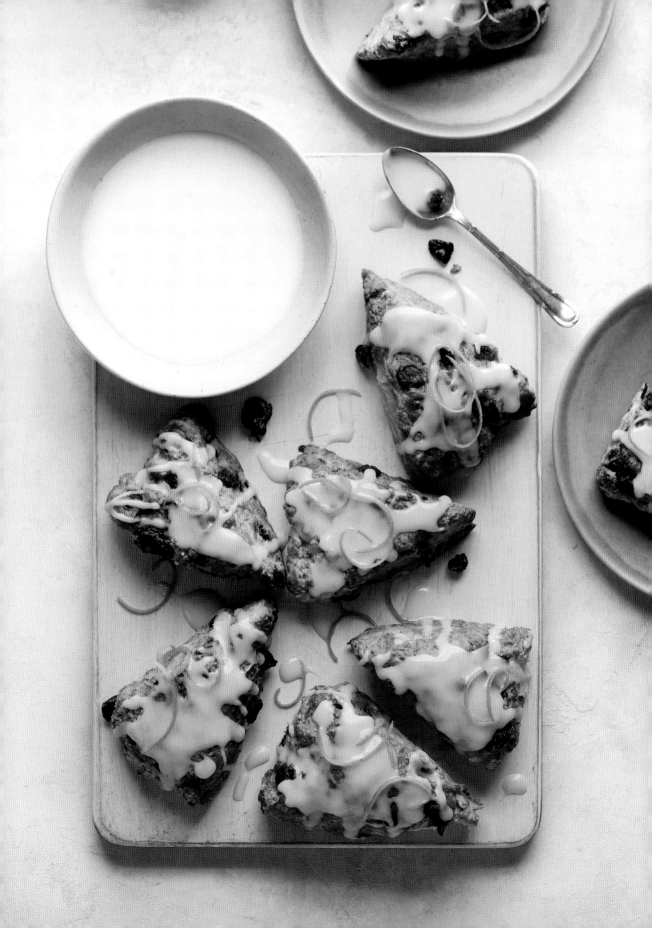

ORANGE, CRANBERRY AND WHITE CHOCOLATE SCONES

190g (6½oz) self-raising flour

1 tsp baking powder

½ tsp bicarbonate of
    soda (baking soda)

pinch of salt

2 tbsp cold unsalted butter

1 tsp orange zest

200g (7oz) fat-free
    vanilla Greek yogurt
    (not Greek-style)

10g (¼oz) white
    chocolate chips

10g (¼oz) dried cranberries,
    chopped into smaller pieces

a little milk, to glaze

For the icing

25g (1oz) icing
    (confectioner's) sugar

a little fresh orange juice

1. Place the flour in a bowl. Add the baking powder, bicarbonate of soda and a pinch of salt and mix well to combine.

2. Grate in the butter and, using your fingers, crumble it into the flours so you have what looks like breadcrumbs.

3. Add in the orange zest and yogurt and fold with a spatula until everything is well combined, then add in the chocolate chips and cranberries.

4. Roll the dough ball around the sides of the bowl to collect any bits that are stuck to the sides, until the bowl is clean.

5. Place the dough on a lightly dusted surface and flatten it out slightly into a circle about 20cm (8in.) in diameter. Cut the circle in half, then in half again. Halve each piece again, until you have created 8 triangles out of the circle.

6. Preheat the air fryer to 180°C/350°F for 2 minutes.

7. Line the air fryer basket with non-stick baking paper or use the grill pan insert.

8. Add the scones, brush over the top with a little milk and air-fry for 10 minutes. Leave to cool.

9. While the scones are cooling, make the icing. Mix the icing sugar with orange juice (just add ½ tablespoon of juice from a fresh orange at a time until it's a drizzle icing – not too thick, not too thin).

10. Drizzle the icing over the top of the scones and serve.

KCALS per serving 154 FAT 3.9g SAT FAT 2.3g CARBS 24.2g SUGARS 5.9g FIBRE 1.1g PROTEIN 5.1g SALT 0.62g

BISCOFF TORTILLA CANNOLI WITH RASPBERRIES

1 Lotus Biscoff biscuit (cookie)

1 tsp brown granulated sweetener

1 low-calorie 20cm (8in.) tortilla wrap (white is best)

1 tbsp Biscoff spread

olive oil spray

about 30g (1oz) light aerosol cream

10 raspberries

Tip

Don't fill the cannoli with the cream until just before eating. If you fill it too soon, the aerosol cream may deflate into liquid.

1. Crush the Lotus Biscoff biscuit into fine crumbs (as fine as you can get) in a ziplock bag. Remove the crumbs, mix with the granulated sweetener and set aside.

2. Using a 9cm (3½in.) biscuit cutter, cut 5 circles out of the tortilla. (Place the biscuit cutter as close to each circle as possible to make sure you get 5 circles – the last one may have a slightly rough edge, but it will still work fine.)

3. Make 5 rough sausage shapes from some foil (these are just to keep the shape of your cannoli, so you don't want them too big or too small).

4. To make the cannoli shapes, roll each tortilla circle around the foil. Secure both ends of the tortilla with a wooden cocktail stick that pierces through both the tortilla wrap and into the foil.

5. Preheat the air fryer to 180°C/350°F for 2 minutes.

6. Line the air fryer basket with non-stick baking paper or use the grill pan insert. Spray with olive oil spray. Spray the cannoli shapes, then place them on their sides in the air fryer basket and air-fry for 5 minutes. Turn the cannoli for the last 2 minutes of cooking.

7. Remove the cannoli shapes, leave to cool slightly, then remove the cocktail stick and foil in the centre.

8. Melt the Biscoff spread in the microwave at 5-second intervals until runny.

9. Dip one end of a cannolo into the melted Biscoff and then dip into the Biscoff crumb. Repeat with the other 4 cannoli.

10. Drizzle any remaining Biscoff spread over the top and sprinkle with any remaining crumb.

11. Carefully place the nozzle of the light aerosol cream into the hole of the cannoli and fill with the cream, then stuff a raspberry into each end.

12. Repeat with the other 4 cannoli and enjoy!

KCALS per serving 74 FAT 2.9g SAT FAT 1.2g CARBS 10g SUGARS 2.9g FIBRE 1.4g PROTEIN 1.2g SALT 0.09g

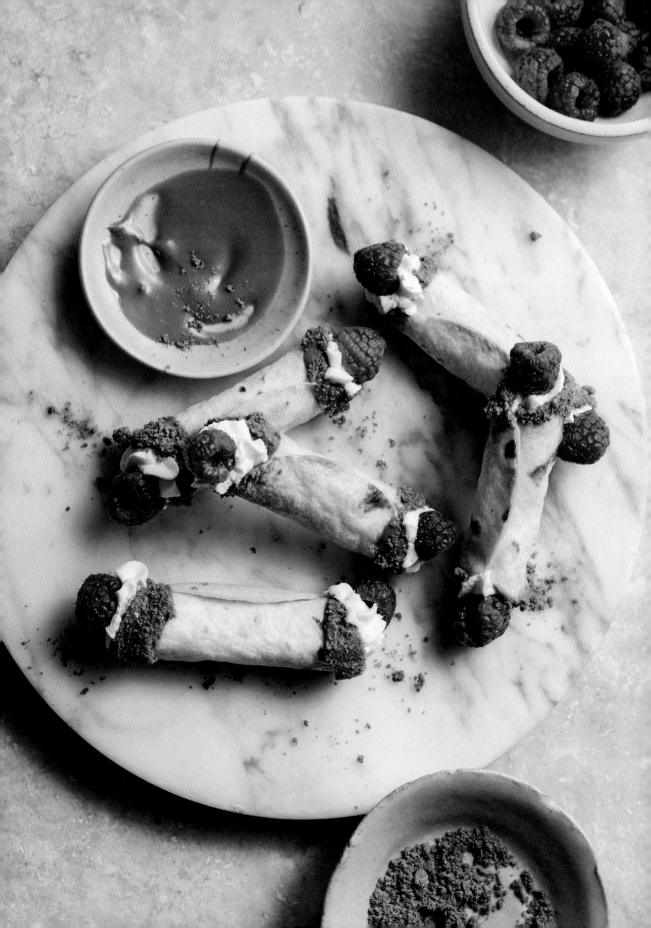

90g (3oz) plain (all-
  purpose) flour
1 tsp baking powder
pinch of salt
80g (2¾oz) banana
12g sugar
3 tbsp brown granulated
  sweetener
1 tbsp unsalted butter, melted
1 medium egg, beaten
1 tsp vanilla extract
40g (1½oz) fat-free
  Greek yogurt

For the maple glaze
½ tbsp unsalted butter
1 tbsp maple syrup
25g (1oz) icing
  (confectioner's) sugar
6g (¼oz) chopped walnuts

MAPLE-GLAZED
BANANA CAKE

1. Mix the flour, baking powder and salt together in a bowl.

2. Roughly mash the banana with the sugar and brown granulated sweetener in a large bowl. Add the melted butter, egg, vanilla extract and yogurt and mix until well combined. Add this mixture to the flour and fold until combined.

3. Pour into a greased rectangular baking dish or foil tray measuring approximately 18cm x 13cm (7in. x 5 in.). Lightly tap the dish on the counter to ensure the batter is distributed evenly in the dish.

4. Preheat the air fryer to 160°C/325°F for 2 minutes.

5. Add the dish to the middle of the air fryer basket and air-fry for 30 minutes, covering tightly with foil for the last 15 minutes of cooking. The cake is cooked when a skewer inserted into the centre comes out clean.

6. Leave the cake to cool slightly, then cut into 6 equal-sized slices.

7. While the cake is cooling, make the maple glaze. Microwave the butter in a small bowl at 20-second intervals (usually a minute in total) until slightly browned (don't burn it).

8. Add the maple syrup and then stir in the icing sugar. Spread over the top of the cake and sprinkle with the walnuts.

KCALS per serving 178   FAT 4.8g   SAT FAT 2.3g   CARBS 29.1g   SUGARS 10.8g   FIBRE 0.9g   PROTEIN 3.7g   SALT 0.33g

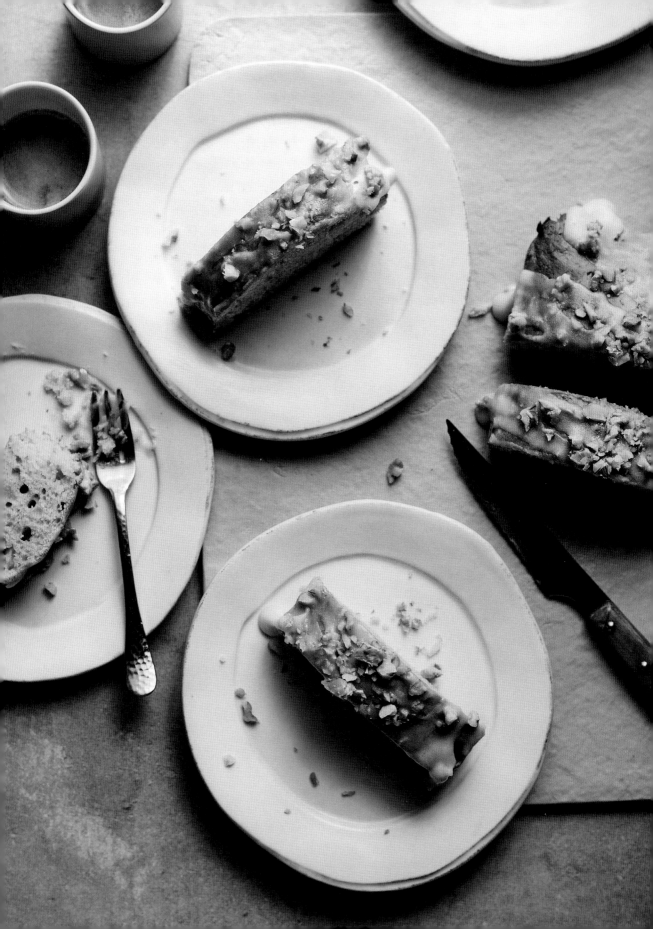

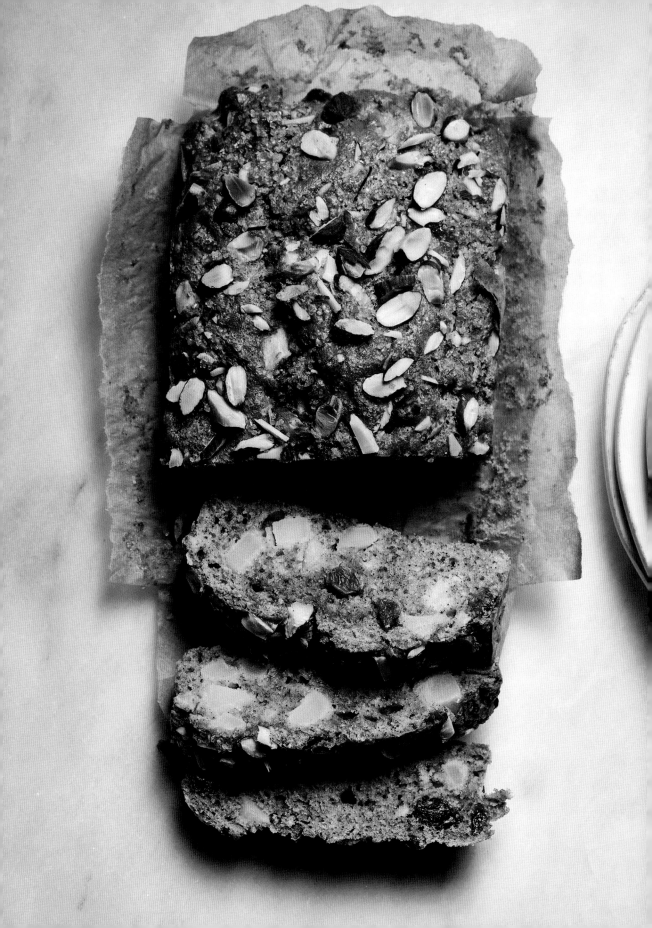

APPLE AND SULTANA CAKE

80g (2¾oz) plain
  (all-purpose) flour
½ tsp baking powder
¼ tsp bicarbonate of
  soda (baking soda)
½ tsp ground cinnamon
pinch of salt
1 tbsp unsalted
  butter, melted
1½ tbsp maple syrup
1 tsp vanilla extract
2 tbsp brown granulated
  sweetener
70g (2½oz) apple,
  peeled and diced
40g (1½oz) fat-free
  vanilla Greek yogurt
1 medium egg
10g (¼oz) sultanas
5g (⅛oz) chopped almonds
1 tsp Demerara sugar

1. Mix the flour, baking powder, bicarbonate of soda and cinnamon with a pinch of salt in a bowl.

2. Add the melted butter, maple syrup, vanilla extract, brown granulated sweetener, apple, yogurt, egg and sultanas and fold together until everything is well combined.

3. Pour into a greased rectangular baking dish or foil tray measuring approximately 18cm x 13cm (7in. x 5 in.), then sprinkle with the almonds and Demerara sugar.

4. Preheat the air fryer to 160°C/325°F for 2 minutes.

5. Add the dish to the middle of the air fryer basket and air-fry for 30 minutes, covering tightly with foil for the last 15 minutes of cooking. The cake is cooked when a skewer inserted into the centre comes out clean.

6. Leave to cool slightly, then cut into 6 equal-sized slices.

KCALS per serving 134   FAT 3.6g   SAT FAT 1.6g   CARBS 21.1g   SUGARS 6.4g   FIBRE 0.9g   PROTEIN 3.5g   SALT 0.34g

SERVES 6
PREP: **15 MINS**
COOK: **30 MINS**

JAM COCONUT SPONGE

1 large egg
24g sugar
4 tbsp granulated sweetener
90g (3oz) fat-free
   Greek yogurt
1 tbsp unsalted butter, melted
1 tsp vanilla extract
85g (3oz) plain
   (all-purpose) flour
1 tsp baking powder
pinch of salt

For the topping
3 tbsp seedless reduced
   sugar raspberry or
   strawberry jam (jelly)
8g unsweetened
   desiccated coconut

1. Whisk together the egg, sugar and sweetener in a large bowl until well combined. Add the yogurt, melted butter and vanilla extract and whisk until smooth.

2. Mix the flour and baking powder with a pinch of salt in a bowl. Sift this mixture into the wet ingredients and then fold gently until combined. Don't overmix (there may be a couple of very small lumps – this is fine).

3. Preheat the air fryer to 160°C/325°F for 2 minutes.

4. Pour the mixture into a greased rectangular baking dish or foil tray measuring approximately 18cm x 13cm (7in. x 5 in.), and place the dish in the air fryer. Air-fry for 30 minutes, covering tightly with foil for the last 15 minutes. The cake is cooked when a skewer inserted into the centre comes out clean.

5. Leave the cake to cool, then spread the jam over the top and sprinkle with the desiccated (unsweetened) coconut. Cut into 6 equal slices and serve.

Side suggestions
This cake is delicious just as it is, or with a little light cream or low-fat custard.

KCALS per serving 163   FAT 4.1g   SAT FAT 2.3g   CARBS 26.2g   SUGARS 7.2g   FIBRE 1g   PROTEIN 4.5g   SALT 0.27g

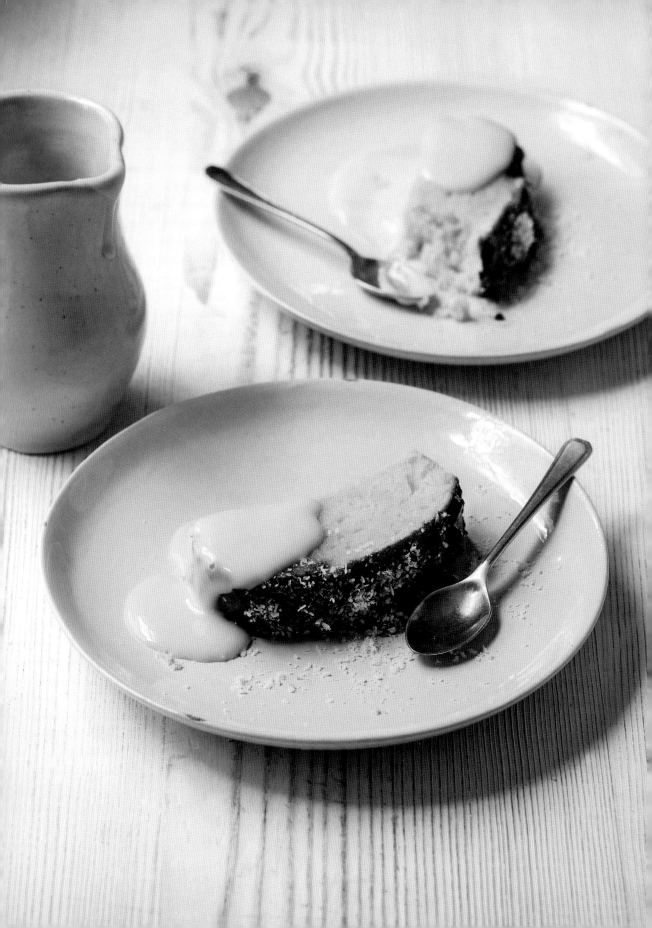

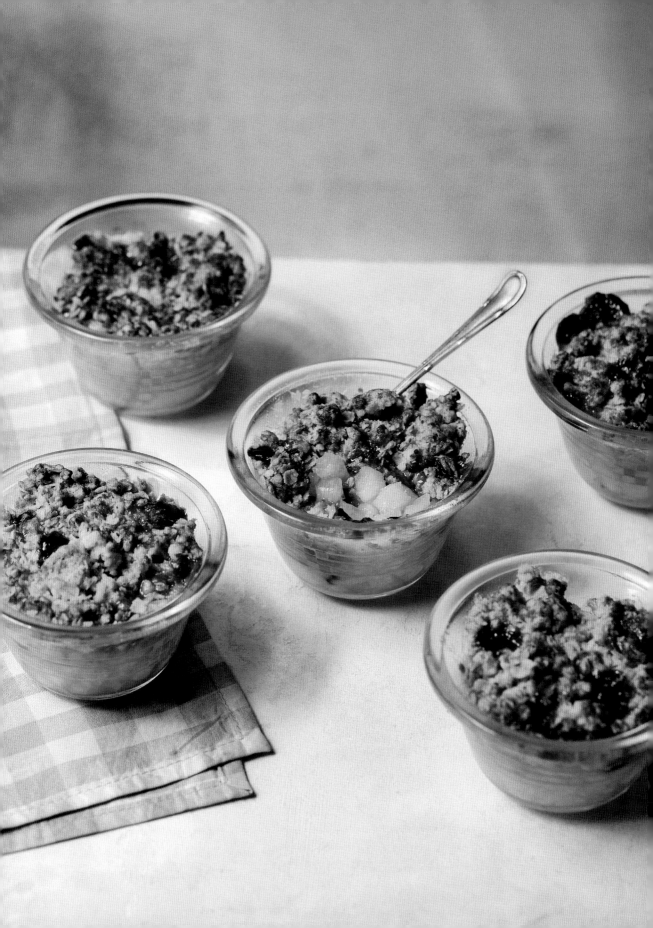

SERVES 6
PREP: **10 MINS**
COOK: **20 MINS**

600g (1lb 5oz) peeled and cored fresh pineapple, finely chopped

6 tbsp granulated sweetener

olive oil spray

1 tbsp cornflour (cornstarch)

40g (1½oz) rolled oats

40g (1½oz) plain (all-purpose) flour

2¼ tbsp desiccated (shredded) coconut (unsweetened)

3 tbsp unsalted butter, melted

1 tbsp golden syrup

32.5g (5 pieces) soft toffees (caramels), finely chopped

PINEAPPLE CARAMEL CRUMBLE

1. Mix the pineapple with 4 tablespoons of granulated sweetener. Place in an ovenproof dish that fits the air fryer basket and spray over the top with olive oil spray.

2. Preheat the air fryer to 200°C/400°F for 2 minutes.

3. Place the dish in the air fryer basket and air-fry for 5 minutes. Mix the cornflour with 1 tablespoon of cold water to make a slurry and add this to the pineapple, mixing until well combined. Air-fry for a further 5 minutes.

4. Divide the pineapple between 6 mini pie cases, distributing it equally.

5. Combine the oats and flour in a bowl with the 2 remaining tablespoons of granulated sweetener. Add the desiccated coconut, melted butter and golden syrup and mix until combined, using your fingers to crumble them into pieces. Fold in the chopped toffee (caramels).

6. Add the crumble mix to the top of the pineapple and spray over the top with olive oil spray.

7. Preheat the air fryer to 180°C/350°F for 2 minutes.

8. Air-fry for 10 minutes until golden on top, then leave to cool slightly before serving.

Side suggestions
Enjoy just as it is or with some light cream or low-fat custard.

KCALS per serving 240   FAT 8.4g   SAT FAT 5g   CARBS 37.4g   SUGARS 14.4g   FIBRE 2.7g   PROTEIN 2.2g   SALT 0.08g

RECIPE INDEX

INDEX

ACKNOWLEDGEMENTS

Well, here we are... at the acknowledgements section of my third book. It's hard to believe and yes, I know I said that in books one and two as well, but it still hasn't fully sunk in!

From a personal perspective, I want to express my heartfelt gratitude to my family – my husband Gavin, and our son and daughter, Isaac and Felicity. They have been actively involved in the testing stage of this cookbook, eagerly waiting to taste each sample as it came out of the air fryer.

I must also thank my dad for always being there and showering me with praise. He probably annoys everyone he meets by proudly talking about his daughter and her accomplishments. Although my mom is no longer with us, I feel her presence and support in everything I have achieved. And to my niece and nephew, Natalie and Danny, sharing every moment of creating this book with you has been incredibly special.

A special mention goes to my friend Kathy. We didn't have as many shopping trips and outings this time around due to my busy schedule, but whenever I needed an escape, you were there for me, as always.

And of course, I want to acknowledge my dear friends Clare, Kerry, Nicky, Nicola and Kate. Despite the distance between us, your unwavering support has meant the world to me throughout this journey.

While it's impossible to name everyone individually, I want to express my gratitude to all my other friends and family who have been supportive over the years.

A big thank you to the fantastic team at Yellow Kite and Hodder for putting everything together on an accelerated schedule. In particular, I would like to thank Lauren Whelan, Liv Nightingall, Miren Lopategui, Alainna Hadjigeorgiou, Callie Robertson, Vickie Boff and Claudette Morris. I'm also incredibly grateful for the exceptional food styling and photography team, consisting of Andrew Burton (photography), Lou Kenney (food stylist), Charlie Philips (prop stylist) and Abi Hartshorne (design).

I want to extend my thanks to Moira, Andra and Steph for their ongoing support of my Facebook community.

Lastly, I want to express my deep appreciation to my readers. If you've been with me from the beginning, I can't thank you enough for your continued support and enjoyment of my recipes. If you've only recently discovered me or stumbled upon this book by chance, welcome! Please explore my website and other publications for more great recipes.

Once again, I sincerely hope you enjoy these recipes and the simplicity of air fryer cooking!

First published in Great Britain in 2023 by Yellow Kite
An imprint of Hodder & Stoughton
An Hachette UK company

5

Copyright © Siobhan Wightman 2023
Photography copyright © Andrew Burton 2023

A CIP catalogue record for this title is available from the British Library

Hardback ISBN 978 1 399 72466 1
eBook ISBN 978 1 399 72467 8

Publisher: Lauren Whelan
Project Editor: Liv Nightingall
Designer: Hart Studio
Photography: Andrew Burton
Food Stylist: Lou Kenney
Props Stylist: Charlie Phillips
Production Manager: Claudette Morris

Colour origination by Alta London
Printed and bound in Germany by Mohn Media GmbH

Hodder & Stoughton policy is to use papers that are natural,
renewable and recyclable products and made from wood grown
in sustainable forests. The logging and manufacturing processesare
expected to conform to the environmental regulations of the
country of origin.

Yellow Kite
Hodder & Stoughton Ltd
Carmelite House
50 Victoria Embankment
London
EC4Y 0DZ

www.yellowkitebooks.co.uk
www.hodder.co.uk

Notes

*The information and references contained
herein are for informational purposes
only. They are designed to support, not
replace, any ongoing medical advice
given by a healthcare professional and
should not be construed as the giving of
medical advice nor relied upon as a basis
for any decision or action. Readers should
consult their doctor before altering their
diet, particularly if they are on a set diet
prescribed by their doctor or dietician.
The calorie count for each recipe is an
estimate only and may vary depending
on the brand of ingredients used, and due
to the natural biological variations in the
composition of foods such as meat, fish,
fruit and vegetables. It does not include
the nutritional content of garnishes
or any optional accompaniments
recommended for taste/serving in the
ingredients list.*